Love Fiercely

Lessons from the Dad
of a Special Needs Daughter

By Andrew T. Bodoh

ISBN: 9798305178302
Imprint: Independently published

Acknowledgments and Dedication

In gratitude for those I write about in these pages, and with special appreciation for all who encouraged me in this project, most especially my friend, Jed Conrad.

Dedicated to my wife, who has made this life of loving fiercely a joy.

Contents

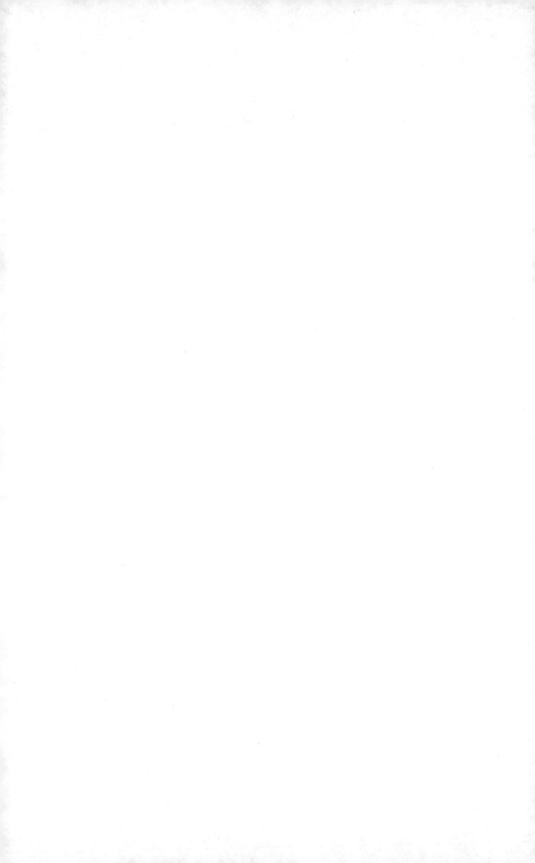

Preface

Dear reader, perhaps you just learned, or at least suspect, that your child will have a lifetime of special needs. I wrote this book for you. Embrace this relationship! Fear and dread may haunt you now. But tomorrow, or tomorrow's tomorrow, will be different, with room for great joy.

Or possibly you are already parenting a special needs child. You and I often don't have words to express to ourselves or others the joy and sorrow, the struggles and delights, shaping our experiences day after day after day. I hope these twelve lessons provide clarity and fellowship, encouragement and strength.

Maybe instead you are the family member or friend of someone parenting a special needs child. You stand outside, looking in. I know you want to be there with and for the one you love. I offer you this glimpse from the inside, to help you cross the divide.

Otherwise, you may be a young man or woman, preparing for the gift of your spouse in marriage. The promises you will make are both fearful and wonderful! Do not underestimate either the challenges of married life or the power of sacrificial love.

And if you are instead a man or woman committed to defending life, know that you are in the prayers of me and my family every day. May God bless you and keep you! And I ask you for your prayers, too, as we work together to share the Gospel of Life.

I Am Not In Control, and That's Okay
Trusting a Loving God

"Goodbye, Elizabeth," I said, with more confidence than I felt. The overnight nurse wheeled my two-year-old away. I clutched my daughter's angel doll as they disappeared through the door, bound for a midnight surgery.

It was a simple brain surgery, if brain surgery is ever simple. Elizabeth has

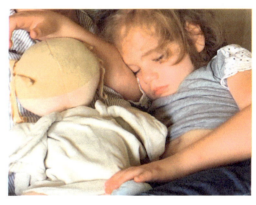

hydrocephalus—that is, excessive cerebrospinal fluid within the skull—from a congenital brain malformation. A pressure valve on the back of Elizabeth's head, under the skin, keeps the fluid from crushing her brain, draining it to her abdomen. But the shunt broke.

Our nanny noticed the symptoms first: vomiting, frequent seizures, and lethargy. Joyce, my wife, sent me a video of this, and I rushed home to Fredericksburg from my law office in Richmond, Virginia. With a backpack of medicine, clothes, and Elizabeth's stuffed angel doll, I drove my girl to her doctors in Charlottesville. Elizabeth slept most of the way—a frightful sleep that left me thinking *Oh God! Child, please wake up!*

We waited in the emergency room lobby for hours. Vomiting, lethargy, and increased seizures don't sound too bad to a triage nurse, compared to strokes and open wounds. But when the chief physician learned of the symptoms, she escorted us through a back door, to a room slated for another patient.

A nurse came in. I answered questions and showed her the video. The ER doctor came in and had me repeat this. The neurology resident came by to ask the same questions and see the video. The neurosurgery team arrived, and I told the story again. Along the way we got X-rays. Then I joined Elizabeth in the narrow confines of an MRI machine. She had to lie still for five minutes as the screeching device imaged her brain, but with her cognitive deficit, she would not do it alone. I lay across her body, propped on my elbows, to comfort her and to hold her face in place.

Later, the medical team tested Elizabeth's cranial pressure more directly. With a hollow needle attached to thin tubing, they poked a small bladder on the subcutaneous valve. We watched yellow fluid rise in the clear tubing, propelled by the high pressure within Elizabeth's skull. By midnight, she was bound for surgery.

Through this all, Elizabeth repeatedly drifted to sleep, holding her angel doll, despite the chaos, and the noise, and her seizures. She woke from a bad bump on the bed as we moved to the pre-op ward. I sat with her as the surgical team prepared. I sang softly as she clutched her angel doll and sucked her thumb. She loved that angel, with its soft body, cotton wings, satin skirt, and tasseled hair.

With the surgeon and anesthesiologist ready shortly before one o'clock, I whispered a prayer, took the angel doll to keep it safe, and said goodbye to my oldest girl.

I briefly called my wife. She was at home with our one-year-old daughter, and I didn't want to keep her up. And after eight hours in the emergency room, I was spent. I could hold myself together when decisions needed to be made, but I was done. I had only to wait, fighting off the creeping anxiety of a nighttime imagination.

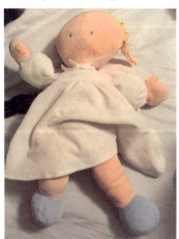

I walked the darkened halls as worst-case scenarios played in my mind. Elizabeth could die. I could get that call, telling me to meet the doctor. He would gently say, "Something went wrong." My daughter could die, and I could do nothing.

Then suddenly, I saw my reflection in the darkened glass of a midnight window. From my backpack, Elizabeth's angel doll stared at me, with her tasseled hair and a smile.

I cried.

In the Gospel of Matthew, Christ says, *"See that you do not despise one of these little ones, for I say to you that their angels in heaven always look upon the face of my heavenly Father."* (Matt. 18:10). Through the kind face of a cotton doll, Elizabeth's guardian angel chided me, telling me I forgot who's in control.

Every night, at bedtime, I recite to Elizabeth the guardian angel prayer:

Angel of God, my guardian dear,
To whom God's love entrusts me here:
Ever this day be at my side,
To light, to guard, to rule, and guide.

Now I lay me down to sleep.
I pray the Lord my soul to keep.
If I should die before I wake,
I pray the Lord my soul to take.

At that moment, in the dark halls of a hospital after midnight, this was the prayer I needed, reminding me to surrender control to a loving God and his angels.

My anxiety sprang from my thirst for control. Anyone with a special needs child knows the feeling. We wish things could be better, even as we fear they will get worse. We are not satisfied doing what we can to improve things. We are too attached to our hopes and fears to be detached from outcomes beyond our control. We fail to separate what we can and should control from what we can't or shouldn't.

The thirst for control creates anxiety. But anxiety cripples our creative powers, becoming self-perpetuating and self-fulfilling. It clouds our imagination, blinding us to the best path forward. And when we act from a place of anxiety, we may damage ourselves and our relationships. Selfishness, intimidation, dishonesty, or even violence may creep in. At the very least, anxiety deprives us of rest. We should be able to rest when we have done all we can do, but the thirst for control demands more. It demands what we can't do. It exhausts us with speculation and self-criticism, and then it feeds on that exhaustion.

Elizabeth's care was out of my hands, and would be for some time. She would need me in the days to come. I should have rested. I should have been able to rest.

But I was imagining a future I could not control. And none of us are good at imagining the future. We see it only in black and white, without the shades of emotional complexity. The good we desire seems greater, and the evil we wish to avoid seems worse than they really will be, and they dominate our focus. The ghosts seem solid through and through, so we pursue phantoms, and dodge shadows.

I needed Elizabeth to be all right. It would break me to lose her—or so it felt. But when I saw the reflection of the angel doll, I knew I needed to surrender control, just as the guardian angel prayer teaches.

The prayer first focuses on relationships, particularly the relationship between me, the angel, and our God. *Angel of God, my guardian dear, to whom God's love entrusts me here.* We cherish our relationship with the angel, our "guardian dear." But this is an angel "of God." God, out of love, entrusted me to this angel—a powerful being who looks on God's face. By entrusting us to his angel's care, God shows us our elevated status. If the angel were to address us, he would call us *a child of God.* He might say, like Gabriel, *"The Lord is with you"* (Luke 1:28), for God made man in his image, marking him as his own. (Gen. 1:26-27). And we been elevated all the more by God becoming man. And God loves us each *personally.* Christ assures us, *"Are not five sparrows sold for two pennies? And not one of them is forgotten before God. Why, even the hairs of your head are all numbered."* Then, in a moment of wry wit, he adds, *"Fear not; you are of more value than many sparrows."* (Luke 12:6-8).

In caring for Elizabeth, I am not alone. I stand in a relationship with a great God who sends her an angel as a guardian. Being in a relationship—truly present *now* at the intersection of *you* and *me*—is the antidote to anxiety. Relationship pulls us from project-oriented thinking, the seedbed of anxiety.

Scripture shows us what a relationship with an angel means. Abraham, Daniel, Tobias, Zacharias, Mary, Joseph, the shepherds of Bethlehem, Mary Magdalene, Peter, John, and many others encountered angels. *"Do not be afraid!"* the angels say. (Gen. 21:1-21; Dn. 10:8-19; Luke 1:11-13, 2:1-12; Matt. 28:1-10; Acts 27:1-26). Fear makes sense when we encounter an angel. Nothing could be more disrupting to our projects and goals than the appearance of a supernatural being in our lives. *"Do not be afraid!"* comforts and assures us, gently inviting us into a relationship of trust.

To trust is to believe another is not only well-intentioned, but also competent. Angels are well-intentioned, for they ceaselessly worship the Lord. (Dn. 7:10; Matt. 18:10; Rev. 5:11-12). And they are powerful, capable of destroying cities or speaking the word that renders a man mute. (Gen. 18-19; Luke 1:20). Yet they submit themselves to our prayerful influence, negotiating with Abraham or answering the inquiries of Mary. (Gen. 18:23-33; Luke 1:34-35). They are messengers and helpmates, instruments in the hand of God. They deserve our trust.

When we recognize God's great gift of entrusting us to an angel, we respond with gratitude. Gratitude is recognizing that this good we have is a

4

gift, incarnating someone's love for us. And in praying from this place of gratitude, we make some humble requests.

Ever this day be at my side. God's angel *will* be with us. But this request reminds me to be attentive to the angel's gentle promptings throughout the day. The angel is at my side. I just need to pay attention.

To light, to guard, to rule, and guide. These are not trite niceties. I take "light" to mean the light of the intellect—the capacity to see things clearly as they are, to know the truth. "To guard" addresses our spiritual and physical security—keeping us from harm and evil. I could ask the angels to guard Elizabeth during her surgery. I could ask them, too, to guard me in my distress, for disordered emotions are doorways for temptation. "To rule" means to judge right actions from wrong, by looking on the face of God. To "guide" means to help us select from among the many paths of righteousness with prudence and charity. It means disposing us to do God's will, by choosing the best from among many good options, or doing a difficult task the right way.

Though we direct this prayer to our angel, these requests orient us to Christ. If we ask our angel to light our minds, our angel will use the light of Christ. (John 1:4). When we ask our angel to guard us, our angel will stand with Christ the Good Shepherd, who lays down his life for his flock. (John 10:11). When I ask my angel to rule me, he will judge me by the standards of Our Lord, the final judge. (Matt. 25:31-36). If we ask our angel to guide us, he will guide us to Christ, who is the Way. (John 14:6).

We parents of special needs children should embrace these words. All children are unique—ours are just more so. We know what it is like to have no answers. We know what happens when the body or brain doesn't work as it should. We know frustration and exhaustion. We know about making best guesses about important things. We know anxiety. And this prayer, asking our angel to light, to guard, to rule, and guide, reminds us to seek the help of God and his angels in our times of distress.

The next lines gently invite our complete surrender to God's will.

Now I lay me down to sleep. To sleep is to surrender. We surrender our minds, our wills, our senses, and our consciousness. We surrender our time. We surrender to our vulnerability, our frailty. We surrender today, for the hope of tomorrow. Surrender is the opposite of control.

If we weren't so hardwired to sleep, some might avoid it completely. If it weren't necessary, sleeping would take an act of faith. But sleep imposes itself on us. And so we accept it, often without recognizing it for what it is: a weak and imperfect foreshadow of death.

We are mortal creatures. We are going to die. When we think of being dead, we often think of it as sleep. We see sleep as an analogy for the experience of death. Even Christ saw it this way. (Matt. 9:24; Luke 8:52; John 11:11). Death is the long sleep, and sleep is like a little death.

In preparing to sleep, then, we practice the detachment we need to prepare for the moment of death. After all, when we go to sleep, we may not awake.

I pray the Lord my soul to keep. At some point, whoever translated this prayer chose rhythm and rhyme over intelligibility. This line might be translated into plain English as, "I hope to God to stay alive." It is about life and death. But the words chosen add something, even with its forced syntax.

"I pray." We only pray to God for what might not come. We pray when something is not entirely within our control. And we are not in control. Life is not guaranteed. I might not be alive tomorrow, so I pray tonight that I will be.

"The Lord." God might be addressed by many titles, but calling him "the Lord" emphasizes his authority over us, his power over our circumstance, and our duty of submission to him. "I pray the Lord" reflects our reliance on God to achieve what we desire.

"My soul." The intimacy of this expression reflects the sincerity of the request. All we value most in life is captured in these words.

"To keep." "Keep" is such an unassuming word. It doesn't have the legal connotations of a word like "possess." "Keep" avoids any hint we have a legal or moral right to our soul vis-à-vis God. I simply ask our Lord for the gift of my soul another day.

"I pray the Lord my soul to keep." The simple language allows the prayer to burst from the soul. We ask God to give us life another day! This urge to live is praiseworthy. St. Paul writes in his Letter to the Romans, *"For if we live, we live to the Lord, and if we die, we die to the Lord. So then, whether we live or whether we die, we are the Lord's."* (Rom. 14:8). This is true, but openness to God's will doesn't require indifference between life and death. Ordinarily, life should be our strong preference, second only to doing God's will.

If I should die before I wake, I pray the Lord my soul to take. Catholic devotionals constantly remind us of death. Our crucifixes depict Christ at the moment of his death—the moment of our redemption. Our Hail Marys ask the Mother of God to intercede for us in the hour of our death. And this prayer, as we end our day, contemplates the possibility of our imminent death.

6

In faith and hope, we ask God for the grace of a good death—a death in which we do not fall away from God, a death in which he receives us into his embrace. Through trust in God, we can face the possibility of death with courage and resolve. We can live without fear of death, accepting the risks of life boldly, without intimidation.

These few lines say so much so simply: *Now I lay me down to sleep. I pray the Lord my soul to keep.* I prefer life! I want to live! I ask God to let me live! *But If I should die before I wake, I pray the Lord my soul to take.* The resignation—the acceptance of our mortality, the possibility of our death—comes with this simple "if," without compromising or undermining the desire for life!

This is how we surrender control: We seek with passion the good, while remaining fully resigned to the will of God! It is nearly a paradox. How can we seek the good with detachment? But our God is a loving God, and he wills only what is good. And so we can pursue the good with courage, enthusiasm, and ferocity if we must, trusting that if the Lord places us on a different path, or if he demands an accounting of our life tonight, he knows what he is doing, and he acts with love. Our passion for the good is secondary to our love of God.

That night, when I saw the reflection in the dark window of that guardian angel doll smiling from my backpack, I had to surrender control. I saw Elizabeth wheeled away, about to go under general anesthesia. *Now I lay me down to sleep.* She needed this surgery. She would die without it, and I wanted her to live. *I pray the Lord my soul to keep.* But things could go wrong, and I had to accept that possibility. *If I should die before I wake, I pray the Lord my soul to take.*

Elizabeth was without me, but she was not alone. *Angel of God, my guardian dear, to whom God's love entrusts me here: Ever this day be at my side, to light, to guard, to rule, and guide.* I may have taken her angel doll, but her angel was still at her side, communicating with the angels of the surgeon, the anesthesiologist, the nurses in the room, and communicating with my angel, through a reflection in the window, to tell me, "Don't be afraid. We got this."

I am not in control…and that's okay. I have the support of a loving God, with a team of angels far more powerful than me.

We must not cling to our thirst for control. As a litigation attorney, I deal with people who suffered trauma. I have seen people driven to psychosis if they cannot detach from control. Their brains become so hardwired to avoid another trauma that they stand on a hair trigger, with their mind constantly alert, seeing in innocent occurrences the possibility of further harm.

7

But every time we think we have conquered the need for control, we find ourselves frustrated, or angered, or frightened, or anxious because of something beyond our control. Elizabeth goes through behavioral cycles, trying to express her needs or soothe her pains by biting, tearing, vocalizing, grinding her teeth, or seeking other stimulation. Her cognitive deficiencies make it difficult to teach her better behaviors, placing them often beyond our control. But every time she grinds her teeth, some part of my brain jerks alive and shouts, "No! Stop! That's not good!" And yet she grinds and grinds and grinds and grinds and grinds, until I beg her to stop. But she grinds on. I cannot control it, but my brain will not surrender my thirst for control. And so I try to form the habit of saying a prayer to her angel, asking for help. And she grinds again.

We are not in control. We want control because it promises us freedom from distress. It promises to expand our world. But we are bad at being in control. We have such a tiny capacity for control that we overreach, and then our thirst for control is controlling us, damaging our relationships and shrinking our world.

We forget what we lose when we grasp for control. Vulnerability, not control, teaches us to trust—to rely willfully on the competence and good intentions of another. Vulnerability, not control, teaches us resilience—to cope with adversity so that we can return to something like the life we enjoyed before the trauma. Vulnerability, not control, teaches us gratitude—to delight in what we have, and in the relationships those things represent, because we know they did not have to be part of our life. We sacrifice these things—trust, resilience, and gratitude—for the illusory promise of control. By seeking control, we confine ourselves to suspicion, obsession, and selfishness. We create the distress that we wish to avoid.

Our model for surrendering control is Christ:

> *Christ Jesus,*
> *Who, though he was in the form of God,*
> *did not regard equality with God something to be grasped.*
> *Rather, he emptied himself,*
> *taking the form of a slave,*
> *coming in human likeness;*
> *and found human in appearance,*
> *he humbled himself,*
> *becoming obedient to death, even death on a cross.*
>
> *Because of this, God greatly exalted him*
> *and bestowed on him the name*

that is above every name,
that at the name of Jesus
every knee should bend,
of those in heaven and on earth and under the earth,
and every tongue confess that
Jesus Christ is Lord,
to the glory of God the Father. (Phil. 2:5-11).

If we were to define perfect control, we could not do much better than saying it is equality with God—the power to bring any result about. That is what the Son possessed. Yet the Son knew control was not *"a thing to be grasped."* Instead, he embraced vulnerability and humble detachment out of love for each of us. This scriptural song highlights the depths of Christ's detachment: He became a servant, like an angel is a servant. Even more, he became a man. Not only that, he submitted himself to death. And not to a glorious death, but to being publicly tortured to death as a reprehensible criminal, with the agonies of the cross. Nailed at his hands and his feet, he entirely surrendered control.

Yet through this submission, Christ won our redemption. *"Therefore God has highly exalted him and bestowed on him the name that is above every name, so that at the name of Jesus every knee should bow, in heaven and on earth and under the earth, and every tongue confess that Jesus Christ is Lord, to the glory of God the Father."*

Control promises us joy through freedom from distress. We will not be vulnerable if we are in control. But relationships require us to accept vulnerability. Relationships require us to lean in and connect with others. In relationships, we are vulnerable because the relationship might end. The other person could break off the relationship. Or the person could die in a midnight surgery, as you wander the halls of the hospital longing for control. But only in and through these relationships do we find joy. Vulnerability, then, is the cost of joy.

I am not in control, and that's okay.

About 3 a.m., my phone rang. The surgery was over. Elizabeth was fine. I returned to the surgical ward, and a nurse led me to the lone patient, my beautiful girl. She was asleep, with a bandage on her head. I delivered to her her angel doll. As the night passed away, I sat with her in the company of the nurses, talking and singing quietly. I called my wife again to tell her we would be alright.

Lesson Two

Sing in Public
Helping Others Encounter Your Child

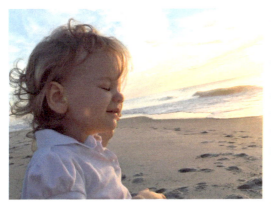

My Elizabeth is so beautiful. She has brown eyes like her mother, a prominent cleft chin, and cheeks made for smiles. Her hair dances on the line between blonde and brown, so thick it defies order. She's inherited my gene for height, sitting above the 97th percentile. We may have named her after the *Pride and Prejudice* heroine.

Elizabeth has a congenital brain malformation. The human brain has four fluid-filled cavities, called ventricles. Elizabeth's are too large, extending to the skull. This is bilateral open-lip schizencephaly. It causes the hydrocephalus. This malformation prevented some brain cells from migrating correctly in utero, producing periventricular nodular heterotopia, which causes seizures. Elizabeth's seizures usually come as a series of spasms. Her arms snap forward and her body jackknifes at her waist. We came to expect these daily, until suddenly, after six years, we found the right medication and they nearly disappeared.

Also, Elizabeth's eye nerves did not develop correctly, severely limiting her vision. This is called septo-optic dysplasia. She can see some light and probably some movement, but very little. Rapid involuntary eye movement, called nystagmus, accompanies this condition.

The brain malformation also impairs Elizabeth's control of her muscle tone, a condition called cerebral palsy. She suffers involuntary muscle contractions, called dystonia, and high muscle tone, called spasticity. In an unmedicated state, she planks her body. She struggles to bend her knees when standing, so she hasn't learned to walk. She uses a wheelchair instead, though with vision and cognitive deficits, she has not learned to push it herself.

Moreover, one of the fluid-filled cavities sits where Elizabeth's speech cortex should be. She uses only rudimentary sounds. If she is happy, she may let out gasps of air and an "Awh!" If she feels prolonged discomfort, she will announce it with loud "Ahhhs." She may entertain herself by blowing raspberries or murmuring "Mum, mum, mum." She seems to hear most language as white noise.

But for all that, Elizabeth loves music. When she hears a song she knows, her eyebrows raise, and her eyes widen. Her hands go up to engage the world, and she stomps her feet. She may dance, throwing her head back and forth with a huge smile.

Elizabeth can enjoy music because it engages many parts of the brain. And through her music skills, she enjoys prayers and has a memory for voices. Her Grandmother and her Aunt Carrie live several hours away, and Elizabeth may go months without being with them. But with the simplest "Hello, Lizzie" from them, she shows all the signs of joy.

Elizabeth also seems to understand intention. She seems to know the difference between someone singing with her present and someone singing to her. This may be extraordinary, but the human brain is not like a computer that stops when it breaks. It is more like an orchestra. If the violin section stops playing, the rest of the ensemble may continue, bringing out sounds overmatched by the strings. Likewise, when part of the brain does not work as it should, quieter operations may make themselves known.

I don't know exactly what Elizabeth's experiences are like, but I have seen too much to believe it is wholly empty, shallow, or bleak. She sits for long stretches without making a sound, just listening, and feeling, and listening. She loves cuddles. She seems to care when Joyce or I are not there to say good night.

But her experiences are different than mine. If I go to a grocery store with her, I see the aisle of food, with each item designed to draw my gaze. I know the olive oil is from Italy, a place far away. I understand the connection between being here now and the meal I will eat tonight. I talk to the people I know. Elizabeth, on the other hand, feels the bumps of her wheelchair as it rolls along. She hears a cacophony of indistinguishable noise. She sees nothing of interest, just a vague blur passing by. She grows bored, tired, uncomfortable in her chair. She lives in a world with little context.

And so I sing to her in public. I have only a small repertoire of songs, much to the chagrin of my wife. There is "How Much Is That Doggie in the Window," made famous by Pattie Page. There is "Red Is the Rose," a song I learned in college but relearned for Elizabeth. I can start a song about raindrops and decide if they are on roses, or if they keep falling on my head. Singing entertains Elizabeth and soothes her.

I take my three girls grocery shopping nearly every week, for some daddy-daughter time. The two younger girls join me as I sing. Becky, at five, knows all the words. She is the extrovert. Marie, at two, is more introverted, but she still throws out the last word of each line. Doe, a— "DEER!" Ray, a drop of golden— "SUHHN!"

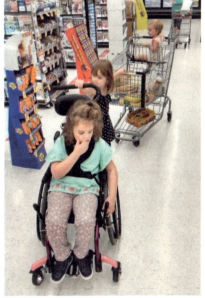

It is a strange and wonderful thing, to walk through a store as a dad, pushing one daughter in a wheelchair, my five-year-old pushing the cart, and the two-year-old toddling behind, singing of raindrops and roses and doggies and tails.

Setting aside my long-suffering wife, most people enjoy the singing. When I sing songs from *The Sound of Music*, strangers will join in, or finish the line if I get distracted. When I crone "How Much Is That Doggie in the Window," someone inevitably remarks she hasn't heard the song in years.

When I sing to my girl in public, I defy social expectations. Singing in public is against the rules. It's not normal. It's embarrassing, or at least that is what I am told. It's a challenge to social conformity.

Society constantly tells us what to think and what to do. It tells us through advertising and stories, laws and policies, and through the way we are treated when we step out of line. It even tells us acceptable ways of defying social expectations. If I wish to be different, I can dye my hair an unnatural shade, or get a body piercing or a tattoo. I can change my pronouns or declare my identity, and demand conformity with my worldview.

Well, society also tells people to ignore my little girl. She's different. She has special needs. Her condition is not contagious, but people don't know what she wants or what she needs, and society says it's impolite to ask—it's impolite to notice her special needs. They are afraid of doing something wrong, and afraid to ask the right thing to do. These are good-hearted people confronting an unusual situation, and they haven't learned how to respond. To avoid offending, they ignore Elizabeth, often even as they engage my other daughters. I have done the same to others. Though I am a parent of a special needs child, it takes effort to connect to someone with special needs.

People will sometimes make an effort, for better or for worse. I often hear, "She must be tired." This tries to express recognition and sympathy, but it still annoys me. Elizabeth appears tired because she doesn't engage sights and sounds around her, because she is nearly blind and cannot process language. So the comment unintentionally points out her deficits. Your first impression of what a special needs child is experiencing is probably wrong. We can do better.

Others engage Elizabeth with physical touch, such as patting her head. Again, this is well intended. But many conditions make simple touches painful or disturbing. Elizabeth's scalp is extremely sensitive, and this is commonplace with cerebral palsy. Strangers don't recognize her signs of distress when they pat or caress her head.

Then there are questions. Personally, I embrace questions. People often must move from disgust or anxiety about the unknown, to curiosity, to acceptance, before they can reach a place of connection. Questions facilitate that. But not everyone feels the same. Questions can seem offensive or demeaning. I give people the benefit of the doubt, but questions are much safer if they rest on a foundation of mutual trust. Please, though, don't scold your child for asking about my daughter, as that only teaches your child to avoid children who are different.

Then there are those who say hello and use Elizabeth's name. This shows true effort, and in most cases, it is great. I don't know that it does much for Elizabeth, as she may not process the voice, but I can't criticize the kindness.

But the truly classy people get to know Elizabeth: The teenager who always converses with Elizabeth one-on-one. The friends who ask how to make their deck more wheelchair friendly. My sister-in-law, teaching her sons to wait for the accessible bus with us. Or our wonderful nannies, who have captured Elizabeth's heart.

The best thing someone can do, when they don't know what to do, is to ask the best way to connect with the child. If you would ask me this, I would say by song. And if you then went to Elizabeth and sang to her in public, you would be a hero in my book, and you would make the day for my little girl.

Encountering children with special needs in public may be the first step toward reducing our fear of childhood disabilities. The expectant father or mother says, "All I pray for is ten fingers and ten toes." This prayer seems humble and modest. Boy or girl, blue-eyed or brown, blonde or brunette doesn't matter. But please God, don't send me a child with special needs. Again, the prayer is well intentioned. But when we accept such social clichés, we reinforce an attitude that matters. This attitude defines the child by her health status and promotes the habitual response of "Thank God it's not me. Thank God my children are healthy."

This attitude matters because it shapes our behavior, it shapes our society. As long as a disability is a bad break for someone else, an unlucky draw, I don't have to think about it. I will use the accessible restroom or park in the handicap spot for convenience. We will put the wheelchair entrance in the back of the store or restaurant, instead of the front. We will minimally comply with ADA laws—maybe—so we don't get sued. We will consider social security programs like Medicaid a waste of money, or burden them with regulations and supervision, or promise a lot and blame the other side when little comes through, because we can afford to.

These things matter. Without a handicap parking spot for my daughter, I would have to leave Elizabeth in a driving lane as I get the other children out of the van. She would not see the car that hits her. She would be strapped to the chair when it crashes to its side.

Or in a public building, look at the barriers between you and an accessible restroom. At one car dealership in Fredericksburg, the restrooms lie in a hallway set about four feet above the main floor, with a wheelchair lift in the far corner of the oversized waiting room, a proverbial mile from the reception desk. My wife once saw chairs blocking the lift. She spoke to the manager. It wasn't a problem, he said, because they didn't mind moving the chairs if someone needed the lift. He was sincere and well intentioned, and before my wife left, he thought better and had the staff move the chairs. But let's play the scenario out anyhow. Many conditions that limit mobility also impair bladder control and continence. A wheelchair user trying to live with a modicum of independence may find herself in urgent need of a restroom. She would spot the restroom sign near a door sitting above a half-flight of stairs. Her access, by a lift, is blocked by chairs. If there were no able customers in the area to help, or if she were too anxious or embarrassed to ask, she would have return to the reception desk. The associate may be occupied with a customer, or may say he cannot leave his post. He may need to call someone to move the chairs. Once the woman makes it back across the room, and the chairs are moved, and the lift takes her up to the higher level, she can make her way down the hallway to the restroom, where she may just find someone using the accessible stall for the convenience of having more room.

If you ask most people without special needs where the problem began, they would identify the chairs in front of the lift. But some architect somewhere decided it wasn't a problem to have the accessible bathroom in a hallway above the main floor. Why? Why make a wheelchair user reliant on a lift to use a restroom? What if the lift breaks? But society tells us stairs are okay, because everyone can climb stairs, or most everyone anyhow, and a lift will solve the problem. And the service desk is far removed from the lift, because there is no connection between the two. And chairs get placed in front of the lift, because it isn't used often, and we can always move the chairs. A series of "No problems" quickly become a significant inconvenience. It's not simply the disability that prevents the woman from using the restroom. It's the assumptions society makes that people won't be disabled. We can do better, and we will do better if we truly encounter those with special needs.

And so I sing in public, so others can encounter my daughter. But I sing for another reason as well. I sing so people will not pity my daughter. Our society pities those with special needs, especially children. A child's suffering is tragic, so the disabled child embodies a living tragedy. Pity is the converse of envy. With pity, the *person who has* feels the *person who has not* should feel deprived. Pity should be reserved for fools, for those who have willfully rejected a spiritual good. It has no place in dealing with those with special needs, for it looks at the person solely as a *has not*, as someone who should feel deprived, as though the disability should dominate the person's consciousness and dictate his mood. Compassion or empathy—entering into the suffering—are appropriate, but pity is not.

The greatest antidote to being pitied is expressing joy. When I sing to Elizabeth, people see the girl in the wheelchair, with her dad and her younger sisters all singing along, and they see her stomping and throwing her head from side to side, and smiling, and smiling, and smiling. The joy radiates forth, affecting those around us. A person who sees joy in Elizabeth cannot pity her. Joy forces the person to reevaluate his perception. It invites him past her limitations, where he might begin to encounter her. We are not supposed to sing in public, and little blind girls in wheelchairs are supposed to be pitied. But you can't pity someone who is full of joy. Social perceptions have to change to account for it.

To encounter Elizabeth and others like her is to be changed. With the encounter, we can set aside our fear of childhood disabilities, our temptations to pity, and replace them with understanding. Childhood disabilities are not a tragedy, but a challenge. They are a challenge for the child, for the child's family, and for the child's community. The challenge lies not only in dealing with the physical, emotional, and cognitive limitations themselves—such as the midnight surgery to fix a blocked shunt—but also in addressing the social context of those limitations—like needing a lift to get to the bathroom. And in and despite the challenge, we may find joy.

Scripture doesn't speak of ADA accommodations or Medicaid policy, but it often shows Christ encountering those with special needs. Consider Christ healing the blind man at Jericho, as recorded by Mark:

> *As Jesus was leaving Jericho with his disciples and a sizable crowd, Bartimaeus, a blind man, the son of Timaeus, sat by the roadside begging. On hearing that it was Jesus of Nazareth, he began to cry out and say, "Jesus, son of David, have mercy on me." And many rebuked him, telling him to be silent. But he kept calling out all the more, "Son of David, have mercy on me."*
>
> *Jesus stopped and said, "Call him." So they called the blind man, saying to him, "Take courage; get up, he is calling you." He threw aside his cloak, sprang up, and came to Jesus. Jesus said to him in reply, "What do you want me to do for you?" The blind man replied to him, "Master, I want to see." Jesus told him, "Go your way; your faith has saved you." Immediately he received his sight and followed him on the way.* (Mark 10:46-52).

Bartimaeus, a blind man, the son of Timaeus, sat by the roadside begging. It seems we have the man's name—Bartimaeus. But "Bar-" simply means "son of," and Bartimaeus means "son of Timaeus." So Mark gives us this man's Jewish nickname—Bartimaeus—followed by a translation for Gentiles— son of Timaeus. It is as though the community has lost a sense of this man's real identity. He is simply "that blind son of Timaeus." The community no longer encounters him as a person, but as a disability.

Bartimaeus is a beggar. He has been reduced to garnering his keep by arousing pity. Pity is always demeaning. Society thinks this blind boy of Timaeus should feel deprived by his condition, because he needs a handout. The community does not enter into his suffering. Instead, those who can afford to prove their moral virtue give a coin or two, every now or then, without troubling themselves to encounter the man. His survival, even if it is meager, proves the generosity of the community—at least in the mind of the proud and haughty—for he has earned nothing. He is *what's-his-name*, living on the generosity of others.

On hearing that it was Jesus of Nazareth, he began to cry out and say, "Jesus, son of David, have mercy on me." Bartimaeus, the nameless beggar, sings out in public, defying social expectations. He asks for Jesus to encounter him. He asks for mercy. Mercy is sympathy put into action. It is entering into another's suffering and doing something good about it.

Bartimaeus calls Jesus the *son of David.* This was a messianic title, for David's household was to rule Israel forever. Society expected a son of David would raise Israel from the bondage of its Gentile masters. This blind beggar suggests Jesus of Nazareth is somehow that savior, even though Jesus is not a warrior. It is the blind man who can see.

And many rebuked him, telling him to be silent. But he kept calling out all the more, "Son of David, have mercy on me." Society constantly tells us our place. Bartimaeus, a beggar, surviving on the good will of the community, does not deserve Jesus's attention. Bartimaeus might embarrass the community. These men in the crowd—not a few, but "many"—not only urge Bartimaeus to be silent, but order him to be silent, rebuking him. But he sings out louder.

Jesus stopped and said, "Call him." So they called the blind man, saying to him, "Take courage; get up, he is calling you." Bartimaeus is the one man of Jerico with heart. He doesn't need the encouragement of these men now. If he had their support before, he would not be on this street crying for Christ's attention.

Yet they speak a platitude: *"Take courage."* How often do those with disabilities hear platitudes? Words that echo a sentiment without engaging the experience? *"It will be all right"* or *"Just pray."* These give more comfort to the speaker than the listener, for it exhausts the wisdom of one without approaching the knowledge of the other, and makes the former feel good for finding a solution at no cost. Through a platitude, one imagines he has aided and consoled, without investing in a true encounter.

The crowd orders this man to *get up,* for he needs permission to accept Christ's invitation, at least in the mind of this crowd. Though he has shown that social opinion doesn't matter to him in this moment, society still tries to put him in his place.

He threw aside his cloak, sprang up, and came to Jesus. He sprang up. The language implies a levity to his actions, and perhaps even joy. He threw off his cloak. He stands before the son of David naked. His disability in this community left him a beggar with only a cloak to his name. In faith, and in defiance of expectations, he tosses away this life he has been living, to throw himself on the mercy of Jesus. In this encounter, he will hide nothing; he will withhold nothing; he exposes all.

Jesus said to him in reply, "What do you want me to do for you?" Christ tests the man's faith. Christ does not reveal his identity or power, as though Christ is asking, "Are you sure I am the Messiah?" But Christ's words, in fact, also echo an ancient question, *"Am I my brother's keeper?"* (Gen. 4:9). A less faithful man would have hesitated, or sought some assurance: "I heard a man called Jesus of Nazareth could heal people in need. Are you that man? Can you heal me?"

But Bartimaeus responds differently. He had family, but they are not here. He should be part of this community, a community that knew—or knows—his father. He is an outcast because of his disability, but still he has joy. He may find joy in the folly of others. He has daily faced the challenge of survival as a blind man in the streets of Jericho, with barely a cloak to shield him from the elements, relying on pity, and demeaned by all. And so, from the depth of his experience, from the depth of his soul, in his nakedness he sings out, *"Master, I want to see!"*

Christ grants this humble request, attributing the healing to Bartimaeus's faith. He releases Bartimaeus, allowing him to go on his way, but Bartimaeus follows Jesus.

Bartimaeus challenged social expectations. He challenged the rules of those who disregarded him, those who avoided encountering him. He sang in public to express his joy at the coming of the Messiah, and to ask for sympathy in action. When Christ responds with words meant to test this beggar's resolve, Bartimaeus asks faithfully for his burden to be lifted. And Christ agrees.

Elizabeth likely will never be healed. But I see her joy in music and song. And my singing helps others to encounter her. Through an encounter with her, and with others like her, we may change social expectations; we may change the world. And so I sing in public.

Lesson Three

Love Fiercely
Confronting Injustices

Early in my career as a lawyer, the parents of a special needs child called me. A school employee hurt their son. As a civil rights litigator, I knew how to help, and I took the case. Sometime later, another case like it came along. And another. I built a reputation for taking these cases.

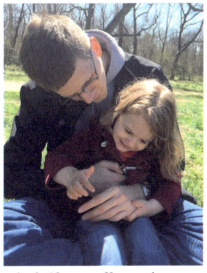

These cases are not common, for many reasons. Special education teachers are usually well trained, and typically have hearts of gold. And the law permits school staff to use proportionate force to protect a student from self-harm, harming others, or from damaging property. And if a staff member acts inappropriately, the parents often will not learn enough of the story to pursue a case. An honest discussion of the economics of litigation also persuades many parents not to sue. The family will need paid professionals to educate the jury about the child's condition and injuries. I will need to be paid. If the child is on Medicaid, the state will need to be reimbursed for the expenses it paid out, with the remaining money put in a trust for the child. I counsel families that keeping their money for therapy and medical treatment is usually better than paying attorneys and experts.

It's no wonder these cases are rare. It's remarkable they happen at all. But they do. Parents of special needs children will sacrifice so much for justice when their child has been harmed. Through these cases, I learned something about these parents. They are fierce.

Then I had Elizabeth, and I understood.

Being fierce is not the same as being aggressive. Fierceness lies in a resolute determination to oppose another, even at a high personal cost. Fierceness is Moses, standing before the Pharaoh, unprotected from his wrath, saying, *"The LORD says, 'Let my people go.'"* (Cf. Ex. 7:16). It is Samson, chained between two pillars, summoning his strength for a mighty shove. (Jdg. 16:23-31). It is David threatening the armored giant, *"Come here to me, and I will feed your flesh to the birds of the air and the beasts of the field."* (1 Sam. 17:44). It is Christ, standing in the wreck of the money changers' tables, saying as he points to his body, *"Destroy this temple and in three days I will raise it up."* (John 2:19).

Put another way, fierceness is anger alloyed with the habit of self-sacrifice. Anger is our natural response to something we see as unjust. When anger moves us to resist injustice properly, it is good. We must respond prudently and proportionately, and we must use legitimate means to oppose the injustice, but anger may be praiseworthy.

Ferocity differs from mere anger, though. The Internet troll and his ilk may be angry, aggressive, and a bully, but not fierce. The person that slaps a child may be angry, but not fierce. The fierce person is *willing to embrace substantial personal suffering* to remedy the perceived injustice. But merely accepting suffering is not fierceness either. The coward accepts suffering, even in the face of an injustice. Fierceness is a willingness to accept suffering *to resist a perceived injustice.*

In accepting the risk of suffering, the fierce man refuses to be intimidated by threats of pain or discomfort, and refuses to be deterred by another's apathy or obstructions. The more suffering he is prepared to absorb without backing down, the more likely he will prevail. A fierce man will not look for conflicts, but he will accept the conflict if the alternative should not be tolerated.

Parents of special needs children must learn to manage conflict. They must often meet petty injustices with a stubborn determination not to back down, even at personal costs, because their child needs it. Conflicts will arise. And if they occur once, they will occur again.

For instance, dealing with insurance companies often involves conflict. Elizabeth has had up to four different prescriptions at a time for epilepsy—sixteen and a half pills a day. Some medications are so strong we need weeks to wean her on or off the drugs. We must work with the doctor's office, the pharmacy, our primary insurance, and our secondary Medicaid insurance for these medications. These insurance companies demand that they approve the prescriptions before they are filled, and periodically as they continue, because they don't want to pay for unnecessary or experimental care. With two insurances, you need pre-authorization from both of them. If the pharmacy does not stock the drug, it will often wait for the insurance companies' pre-authorization before ordering the medicine.

And so, when Elizabeth's medications run low, I call the pharmacy for a refill. It puts me into an automated phone tree. The options are always new, just like they were last month, so you have to listen carefully. *If this is a medical emergency, hang up and dial nine-one-one. Did you know the pharmacist can now provide many of your over-the-counter medications through the drive-thru? Now what did you call about today? I'm sorry, I can't understand you. Can you say it again in a clear and slow voice? Do you want a prescription refilled? Say yes or press one for yes. Say no or press two for no. Please say or enter the birthday associated with the account using two digits for the day, two digits for the month, and four digits for the year. Let me look that up. All right. Are you Elizabeth? Say yes or press one for yes. Say no or press two for no. Please say or enter the eight-digit prescription number, followed by the pound key. I'm sorry, I didn't get that. Please say or enter the eight-digit prescription number, followed by the pound key. I'm sorry, I didn't get that. Please say or enter the eight-digit prescription number, followed by the pound key. If you don't have the prescription number, press nine to speak with one of our team members. Thank you. Due to staffing shortages, we are experiencing greater than expected hold times. Please hold. We value your business.*

The pharmacist will likely tell me if the prescription has expired, but normally she won't know if the pre-authorization needs to be renewed. Instead, I will get a vague, automated call sometime later, urging me to call the pharmacy for more information. The pharmacy will have me call the insurance company. I prepare for another phone tree. *We value your business.*

When I reach the call service representative, I expect to be told to call my doctor's office. But sometimes it's worse. Maybe they will transfer me to another call center, because the notes indicate the pre-authorization six months ago went through their subcontractor, only to learn after thirty minutes that the subcontract expired five months ago. Or the representative will say the call center only manages the Medicaid pre-authorizations, and I need to call the number on the back of the primary insurance card, even though that was the number I called. Or I will hear the authorization is under review and I need to call back tomorrow, only to learn tomorrow the company rejected the authorization two days before because of a typo and the doctor needs to start over.

This is all frustrating, and when this nonsense leaves me staring at my daughter's last pills, reducing the dose to stretch the supply a little further before she goes cold turkey on a medicine so strong it requires a month of titration, I will be fierce. I will tell you what my situation is, and we will not end this call until there is a solution. And if you hang up, I will call back, again and again. I will document everything. Then I will research the state and federal regulations and report every violation I find to the appropriate government agency, because that will ring your bell. Did I mention I'm a lawyer?

Insurance companies are an adverse side effect that comes with every drug. And that fight occurs again and again. But my fiercest fight involved bringing Medicaid to court after their doctor decided my daughter needed weight management instead of a bathroom.

We learned some years ago that Elizabeth could qualify through Medicaid for up to five thousand dollars toward home modifications. That was great news. Elizabeth's wheelchair wouldn't fit through our bathroom doors. We had no bath or shower on the main floor, no lift for her at the stairs, and no accessible bath or shower upstairs. We would carry our thirty-five-pound two-year-old girl upstairs to bathe her, hoping she would not start seizing on the stairway or in the tub. We planned to cover the extra costs, but Medicaid promised some money for these projects.

We heard stories, though, of other families struggling to get this money. Families dealing with child elopement issues might be denied money for a fence or a video monitoring system. Those with a child dependent on machines might be denied money for a generator. In fact, the money was supposed to be available for vehicle modifications, too, but the state audited all dealers some years ago, revoking money it already paid based on regulatory violations, and now no one in Virginia will do vehicle modifications for Medicaid dollars.

We got no clear guidance on how to apply for funds. But I submitted a detailed narrative, with pictures, medical records, notes from Elizabeth's doctor, and a proposal. Weeks later, Joyce got the call. Our request was denied because the modifications would cost more than five thousand dollars. We pointed out there was no cap on the cost, just a cap on the reimbursement. We would cover the rest. We asked for a written decision, so we could appeal, and that was initially refused. We demanded it, and a week later they sent the letter.

But the letter didn't say the project would cost too much. Now it said the modifications weren't medically necessary. It ignored Elizabeth's cerebral palsy and brain malformation, and minimized her medical condition as merely developmental delays, seizures, and visual problems. It suggested we should use our existing bathroom.

I began the appeal process, learning the legal regulations and tracking violation after violation along the way. For instance, only a basic pediatrician reviewed the initial request, when federal regulations required review by a doctor with clinical expertise in treating Elizabeth's complex medical conditions. Likewise, buried in the regulations, I found we could demand an in-person hearing, and the decision makers for the appeal had to consider any evidence we presented. Of course I demanded it. The company adopted its hearing protocols just one day before I received them. At the hearing, the room was full, but the external physician who would make the decision was not there, and no one recorded my statements. How could the absent decision maker review unrecorded in-person evidence?

Two months after the initial denial we received the decision. The request was denied. The outcome itself did not surprise me. But the rationale angered me. The letter cited peer reviewed medical literature about recovery after strokes or after hip fractures—not about getting a little blind girl with seizures and cerebral palsy a shower or sink. Then the external physician concluded we should use an existing bathroom and a special bath seat, continue therapy, and we should start weight management for an overweight toddler.

Weight management for an overweight toddler? My child is blind. She had daily seizures. She has low cognition. She has cerebral palsy and uses a wheelchair. She would continue to grow. We would still be carrying her upstairs to bathe her. And the long-term solution is weight management? What would this doctor recommend? Yoga, or Pilates?

We appealed again, this time with a letter of medical necessity citing twenty-one medical articles concerning her conditions and their proper care. I showed the prior decisions were based on the wrong body of regulations, and so the hearing officer reversed them. But the process started all over. The same pediatrician denied the request again. I appealed and demanded an in-person hearing. This time they recorded the presentation, but the same external physician denied the appeal. I appealed again. At the next hearing, testimony showed my in-person evidence was not even submitted to the external physician. It didn't matter. A year after submitting the initial request—a year of carrying Elizabeth up and down the stairs for baths, a year of further growth, a year without the chance to teach her even how to wash her hands at a sink—the hearing officer ruled the modifications were not medically necessary. And he bluntly concluded the regulatory violations were outside the scope of the appeal hearing. It was time for the courts to get involved. I appealed again.

But with the courts involved, the Virginia Attorney General's Office took over the case for Medicaid. These are good attorneys. I got a call. After some time, we got a resolution. Medicaid would cover five thousand dollars of the bathroom modification, and by law, it would pay some additional fees for my time as Elizabeth's attorney. And so, two and a half years after we first submitted our request, as Joyce and I went to the hospital to deliver to Elizabeth a second baby sister, a contractor was modifying our bathroom.

I heard rumors that as our case progressed, other families found their requests for modifications being approved without appeal, even after previous denials. I hope so, for I poured hundreds of hours into research, writing, and arguing. We did it for ourselves and these other families.

Every parent of a special needs child will collect similar stories, confronting the schools, the hospitals, insurance companies, or God forbid the justice system. These parents must be fierce. This is an essential competency, usually learned on the job.

But ferocity comes naturally when you are raising a special needs child. These children are prone to suffer injustices they cannot remedy. Parents

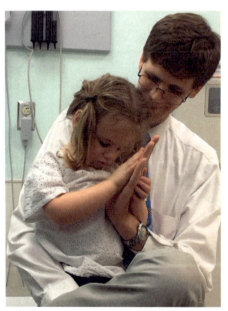

will *see the injustice* and *feel anger.* And the parents' long habit of self-sacrifice—from appointments, to IEP meetings, to in-home therapies, to fights with the insurance companies—means they are *not intimidated by suffering.* It's not that they don't suffer, but rather they will endure it to remedy the injustice. They are fierce.

This fierceness flows directly from love. Love and ferocity operate hand-in-hand. Love means *seeking the good of the other,* while fierceness involves *recognizing an injustice.* Because we seek what is good for our child, we see the injustices they suffer. Love is a *willingness to sacrifice ourselves for the beloved,* and fierceness requires *a willingness to sacrifice ourselves to oppose the injustice.* So love and ferocity both involve a willingness to sacrifice ourselves. Thus, injustice toward the child we love provokes a fierce response. In other words, parents of special needs children learn to love fiercely.

Love is patient, love is kind. We know this. We hear it all the time at weddings. *It does not envy, it does not boast, it is not proud. It does not dishonor others, it is not self-seeking, it is not easily angered, it keeps no record of wrongs.* This seems incompatible with the idea that love is fierce. *Love does not delight in evil but rejoices with the truth. It always protects, always trusts, always hopes, always perseveres.* (1 Cor. 13:4-7). St. Paul describes love correctly, but love is also fierce.

Love is patient. Love is patient toward the beloved, and toward others, but it is not passive. Patience is waiting with a purpose. Patience without purpose is merely passivity. When and injustice must be remedied now, such as when the prescription must be filled, patience cannot abide waiting further. Love requires patience to give way, in some measure, to fierce action.

Love is kind. We can be both fierce and kind. If we reject the option of being passive in the face of pressing injustice, kindness is having a sword available, and responding instead with tact. Kindness in the face of injustice means using the least offensive means possible to oppose the injustice in a reasonable manner. Fierce love can be kind.

It does not envy, it does not boast, it is not proud. These three vices can inspire misguided ferocity—ferocity without love. If we envy another, we may persuade ourselves that we see a real injustice, because *I deserve what they have,* and this may provoke unjustified fierce anger. If we are boastful, we may act fierce for the story we'll later tell, not for the sake of justice. If we are proud, the slightest perceived insult may provoke a disproportionately fierce response. We must avoid this. We must keep our ferocity rooted in love, free from envy, boasting, and pride.

It does not dishonor others, it is not self-seeking, it is not easily angered, it keeps no record of wrongs. These are not easy instructions, but they do not foreclose fierce love. Ferocity, motivated by love of another, tries to stop a real injustice. Once we have achieved that, our anger should cease. We should not act maliciously to destroy the reputation of the other through dishonor, or to gain something extra for ourselves. We should forgive and keep no record of wrongs. I can't say, when it comes to insurance companies, that I have reached that point.

I love that St. Paul says that love is not *easily* angered, because anger is not the opposite of love; it is compatible with love in some way. Anger is love responding to an injustice. We should not be easily angered, because we should try to understand the other point of view, we should respond proportionately, and we should not be aroused by contrived injustices. But anger may be what love demands. We are sometimes called to act fiercely.

Love does not delight in evil but rejoices with the truth. If we take this seriously, we must not take our ferocity an inch too far. Ferocity tends to delight in aggression, in inflicting retributive pain. But if that aggression or pain goes further than it must, it is evil, and we are delighting in evil. Ferocity must be tied to a true injustice for it to be compatible with love. The willingness to sacrifice ourselves must be true, too, and not an excuse for delighting in evil.

It always protects, always trusts, always hopes, always perseveres. These are, I think, the circumstances that may provoke our fierce love. I will *protect* Elizabeth, so you will do no harm. I will *trust* her, so you will sow no seed of doubt. I will *hope* for her future, so you will not tell me to despair. And I will *persevere*, so you will stand down or stand aside.

We parents are called to love our special children, and to love our neighbor. Love seeks the good. But when love encounters an injustice, we will resist. We will suffer if we must. We will be fierce. We are called to love. We are called to love fiercely.

Lesson Four

Live in Mercy
Acknowledging Your Imperfections

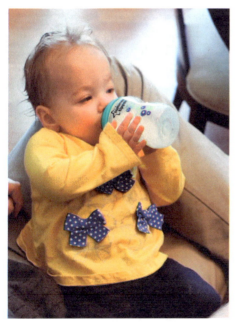

For a few months, before Elizabeth's first birthday, she was almost an ordinary girl. She could hold her bottle and drink her milk. She started to eat solid food. She would sleep well, cuddling her blanket and angel doll, sucking her thumb. She wasn't crawling, but it was only a small delay, we thought. The frantic rush of appointments subsided. Her shunt worked as it should. A video from that time shows a girl with an oval face, sprouts of dark hair, laughing in my arms as I attack her with kisses. We planned a trip to Florida to see space shuttles, and we were open to making Elizabeth a big sister.

We learned Joyce was pregnant days after an emergency hospital stay cancelled our trip to Florida. Elizabeth's epilepsy entered our life without warning, with series of spasms, when she was eleven months old. I stayed with her in the hospital, trying to keep my curious girl from pulling the wires glued to her skull, monitoring her erratic brain.

The visit launched us into the world of antiseizure medication and treatments. It is more like wizardry than medicine. Neurologists evolve drug cocktails like potions to target different aspects of the disordered brain activity, often without knowing why these drugs work. It is practice and error. Keppra caused Elizabeth to be aggressive and irritable. Klonopine didn't work. Sulfa drugs caused hives. The complexities of a broken brain and imperfect science keep us guessing. If the medicine did not make a difference, should we increase the dosage, or move on? If the seizures got worse, was it because of the flu she had, or the medicine change we made last month? At what point is some control over the seizures good enough?

I fortunately don't make many life-or-death decisions for Elizabeth. Some parents face impossible choices. But in a gentler way, managing Elizabeth's medications taught me how to make serious decisions in the face of uncertainty.

You ask the typical questions. *If it works, what would you expect to see? How likely is it to work? What are possible side effects? What are the alternatives? Why is this option better?* This tells me the medical information, but I have to consider the lifestyle implications. We moved Elizabeth onto the ketogenic diet at one point, starving her body of carbohydrates and sugars, because burning fat somehow controls seizures, sometimes, with few side effects. A single slice of bread contained all the carbs Elizabeth could have for the day. The diet worked about as well as the previous medicines. But she started refusing to eat, and whipping together a peanut butter and jelly sandwich was not an option. For a girl with few sensory pleasures and too much pain, the sacrifice eventually did not justify the gain.

Then there was the Cannabidiol oil. This was highly concentrated pharmacy grade stuff, costing far more than my salary for a yearly supply. It worked better than the prior medications. But it was mixed with strawberry-flavored sesame seed oil, which was as bad as it sounds. Elizabeth would purse her lips, so I slipped it in along her cheek. She learned to squeeze those, so I went through a gap in her teeth. She would collect it in her mouth and spit it out. I gave her smaller doses. She refused to swallow it. If we mixed it with something, then everything tasted like strawberry-flavored sesame seed oil, and we had more to feed her. Yet we couldn't waste a drop, or we might run out before we were allowed another refill.

At some point, you realize that you are traumatizing your child—literally causing the child trauma. Often that realization comes long after it should have. It happened again with Elizabeth's hair. Her cerebral palsy makes her scalp highly sensitive. In the shower as I tried gently to undo the tangles in her beautiful hair, she would wail and defend herself by slapping and biting, grabbing my hands or the comb and not letting go. After far too long, I told my wife we had to cut Elizabeth's hair—and cut it short.

Then there are the accidents and oversights that injure your child. Elizabeth will have a permanent scar from the time I stepped away to grab something as she sat on the edge of a hotel bed. I saw her sliding forward and I tried to stop her, but she hit a nightstand, leaving a deep cut.

These are the day-to-day struggles of parents of special needs children. And to mitigate the fights over medicine, the meltdowns, and the risks of injury, we compromise our ideals. If chocolate milk or candy in the morning gets her to take her pills, then we call it breakfast. If she is safe in the recliner, that's where we will leave her for hours at a time. Real life isn't easy. Joyce and I come home exhausted from work to take over for our nanny who is exhausted from work. Instead of exercises or stretches with Elizabeth, we watch television, as she sits in the recliner. We often hear what more we can do for Elizabeth. More therapy. See another specialist. Another piece of equipment to use. More therapy. But instead, she sits in the recliner, because work and life are exhausting.

And this is only one child. We have been blessed with two children more, and a third on the way. Elizabeth teaches her siblings compassion, and they give her help and joy. But then there are more lessons, and more schedules, and more distractions, as Elizabeth sits in her chair.

And with all of this—the questions with no answers, the trauma you cause, the oversights and injuries, the compromises, and the exhaustion— you judge yourself and become discouraged. Your child, your family, and your life aren't where they should be, and it's your fault. You could be doing more.

The truth is, that's probably right. You could do more. You could pay better attention. You could give up your job and cover more therapy appointments. You could hire more help. You could drain your financial and emotional resources to try to get your child to be a little better, or your life a little more in line. But that doesn't mean you should.

Look at your child. Something in the beautiful mechanisms of the human body broke. Her body must compromise, adjust, and make do. Just the same, her family must compromise, adjust, and make do. You must adjust. And just as your child's health is never perfect, and her body can never fully adjust, your family will never fully adjust. Your family will never operate at maximum health. Don't be attached to that goal. You are not in control.

But you love fiercely. You sacrifice so much for your child, fighting this brokenness. Along the way, you make mistakes. You cause your child pain. You step away from the bed and she falls. She resists her medicine and you force it. You make mistakes. And the echo chamber of your mind will amplify every mistake.

31

How often does Christ talk to us about his mercy? What does he say? *"If you forgive others their transgressions, your heavenly Father will forgive you."* (Matt. 6:14). *"Blessed are the merciful, for they will be shown mercy."* (Matt. 5:7). *"Go and learn the meaning of the words: 'I desire mercy, not sacrifice.'"* (Matt. 9:13). Does he prove his mercy? *"For God so loved the world that he gave his only Son, so that everyone who believes in him might not perish but have eternal life. For God did not send his Son into the world to condemn the world, but to save the world through him."* (John 3:16-17). *"[O]ne soldier thrust his lance into his side, and immediately blood and water flowed out. An eyewitness has testified, and his testimony is true; he knows that he is speaking the truth, so that you also may believe."* (John 19:33-35). Christ is the God who became man and literally allowed his heart to be open to us, to show us his mercy.

If Christ extends his mercy to those who practice mercy, and if Christ longs for us to offer mercy and not sacrifice as reparation for sins, we must consider what it takes to show mercy to others. Too often we think of mercy merely as forgiving those who have done us wrong. Scripture presents a much broader vision of mercy. Mercy is sympathy in action. Christ shows mercy through care for those in need, especially those with physical needs. He heals the blind and cures the lepers. (E.g., Mark 1:40-45, 8:22-26; Luke 17:11-19). He subdues the epilepsy of a boy and raised a girl from the dead. (E.g., Mark 5:21-43, 9:17-29). And he wants others to share in that mission. After all, when Christ describes the final judgment, when he describes separating the sheep from the goats (Matt. 25:31-46), he does not apply a rule of "Thou shall not." He instead looks for deliberate and concrete acts of mercy toward those in need: feeding the hungry, clothing the naked, visiting the imprisoned, and the like. Among those acts of mercy, Christ mentions caring for the sick. *For when you do this for the least of my children, you do it for me.* Our daily care for those with special needs is dear to the heart of Our Lord. We are living in mercy.

And Christ knows our imperfections. Just look to the father of the boy with seizures. (Mark 9:17-29). This man clings desperately to hope, feeling the pull of despair, as he sees the sufferings of his beloved child. Yet the Apostles cannot cure the child, and the father pleads with Jesus, *"If you can do anything, have compassion on us and help us."* *"'If you can!'"* Christ responds. *"Everything is possible to one who has faith."* Mark records the boy's father crying out, *"I do believe, help my unbelief!"* And for this prayer, this acknowledgment of frailty and imperfection, Christ extends his mercy.

Christ entrusted this special child to you, and he knows our human frailties. If he loves your child half as much as the Gospels suggest, he will love you for caring for his child through all your sufferings, even with your mistakes. Christ grew thirsty and hungry. (Mark 11:12; John 4:6-7). He grew tired and rested as others around him labored. (Matt. 8:23-27). He needed time alone. (Luke 4:1-2, 14-15; Matt. 14:1-3). When you give so much for your child, whom Christ loves, he will not treat you harshly for those things you presume to be your mistakes.

Live in mercy. Mercy is not simply forgiveness. Mercy is living in relation to a suffering soul. Too often we caregivers judge ourselves by what our child doesn't do: She doesn't walk, doesn't talk, doesn't take her medicine without chocolate milk in the morning. And we blame ourselves for not doing more. Our children will not be judged before God by a footrace or an oral test, much less by a health exam. They will be judged by the standards of love, and they learn love through relationships, not through an extra therapy session. Maximizing your child's relational potential is more important than maximizing your child's physical potential.

And bringing your child into relationship with others may create more distractions from your child's care. If Elizabeth has a sister—or two sisters, and a brother on the way—we will be busy teaching them to walk, to talk, and to engage the world. We have other meals to serve and baths to give, other appointments and other play time. Elizabeth will get less of my time—

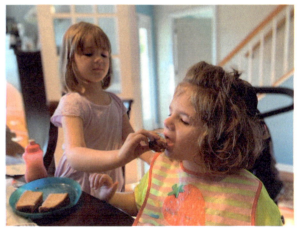

but she gets sisters and a brother. By eighteen months old, my daughters learned to feed Elizabeth. By two, they joined in the songs Elizabeth loves. By three, they pushed her wheelchair, even when they could not see over it. At five, my oldest cared for Elizabeth when we had to step away. What dividends will these lessons of compassion pay in the future, for Elizabeth and her siblings?

Live in mercy. Accept the possibility that you are doing okay, and maybe you are doing the best you can do, and maybe the best is what you are doing. Your worst judgments of yourself are probably wrong. Your child needs you for the long haul, and that means finding time for self-care, and finding a way to let go of your mistakes, real or perceived.

It does not mean you excuse neglect. It means that you accept your frailty and trust in the mercy of God. Raising a child with special needs is not easy. It's hard to be a caregiver. But you are showing mercy to another, and God has promised his mercy in return. Your self-doubt and mistakes do not mean anyone would do better.

Parents do fall into ruts with their children. They know the tablet or television will keep the child quiet, calm, and contained, to avoid tantrums and conflict. This is far too easy with a special needs child, when options are fewer, the burden is greater, and the meltdowns are more severe. Often we don't see the rut until someone points it out. Know this happens to all of us, no matter how much we love our children, and don't judge yourself harshly when it happens to you. God knows there is not enough time in the day. God knows you have limited energy. God knows how easy it is to forget. He made you that way. You are human.

Self-criticism may be a sign you cling too much to something beyond your control. If you cling to what your child should be or do, or what your family should be or do, or what your life should be, you are vulnerable to self-criticism when you encounter your limits.

But I know this is not always the right answer. When your child depends on you to learn what they can do, and when others decide quickly what your child can't learn, clinging to hope and pursuing therapy and specialists and exercises and training is a heroic act. Can we cling to this hope without clinging to control? Maybe, but it is not easy.

Living in mercy must also extend to your spouse and other caregivers. Raising a special needs child will test a relationship, and partners must either lean into each other for mutual support, or the relationship will break. Supporting your spouse often means humbly swallowing your criticisms, and assuming your spouse does the same. It means trusting her good judgment even if you disagree, and keeping a conversation alive if she wants even though you are pretty sure you made up your mind. Joyce and I find that I look at changes cautiously, knowing what we have and concerned we may lose ground. Joyce looks at changes hopefully, seeing the health markers we have not achieved and believing the next treatment will close the gap. If I see a baseline of ten seizures a day, I fear a new medication will increase that to twenty or will have adverse side effects. Joyce hopes the medication will eliminate the seizures and the existing side effects. We may disagree, but we don't argue as we work toward a consensus.

Living in mercy means reframing perceptions. With the first diagnosis or first sign of delay, you will ask, "Did I do something wrong to cause this?" Or "Is God punishing me for something I did?" The answer is usually *No*, but that will not quell the doubts. Reframe the perception. Recognize that God has given us a great intellect, but our minds prefer to invent a story of blame with any unfortunate event. Questioning if you are to blame is an uncomfortable step toward accepting the new reality. You will question yourself, but don't make up your mind that you are to blame. No one needs to be blamed. How things came to be doesn't change what your child needs now, and that must be your focus.

Self-criticism also arises as you try to rebalance your life to accommodate the demands of extraordinary childcare, or when you face an impossible medical decision. No matter what you choose, you will doubt whether you did the right thing. And unfortunately, this is not a one-and-done challenge. You have to rebalance your life again and again and face the medical questions over and over as the conditions develop. Repeat after me: *I made the best decision with the information available at the time. I made the best decision with the information available at the time.* Be deliberate and thoughtful in reaching a decision. Ask questions and study the options. Then make a decision. When doubts arise, as surely they will, drown them out by saying *I made the best decision with the information available at the time.* Judge yourself by the decision process, which you can control, not the outcomes you can't.

You may also criticize yourself when your child acts out in public. But there are only two types of people in this world: those who see your child acting out and accept it, and those who judge you. You don't have to worry about the first type. The second type just needs to learn what a world with special needs children looks like, and your child is teaching them, so you don't need to worry about them either.

This is a glib answer, and I wish it were that simple. Parents struggle to decide what behaviors of their child to tolerate in public and what behaviors to curb. They don't want to be the center of attention or annoy others. They don't want to be judged. But they also don't want the stress of constantly correcting their child or worrying about a sudden outburst. It drains the parents' energy and deprives them of any pleasure in the outing. And that makes them ripe for self-criticism.

I have a beautiful daughter in a wheelchair. Our society smiles at a father but scowls at a mother when their child acts imperfectly. When Elizabeth acts out with me, people generally let it be. Imagine the challenge of a mother whose well-built, teenage son has a behavioral condition instead, such as oppositional defiant disorder. When he acts out, the public sees an ordinary boy acting inappropriately. She gets no benefit of the doubt.

I can only think of two things to say to that mother, and neither provides much consolation: It's a hell of a thing, and remember that Christ was misjudged, too. I don't think it's irreverent to say those two together. Christ was misjudged and suffered a hell of a thing to save us. After all, he was battling the forces of hell, and we were the prize. The suffering of that child, through his behavioral disorder, and the suffering of that mother, make up what is lacking in the sufferings of Christ. (Col. 1:24). Christ will not forget their sufferings.

But for the sake of that mother and her son, I will sometimes let my daughter sing in public. I will let her express herself in the language God has given her—in her claps and her moans and her kicking. If our society sees this, then maybe—just maybe—our society will be a little less judgmental, a little more willing to assume that others are doing the best they can, no matter their physical or behavioral limitations.

God will have mercy on us for our mistakes. But as a Catholic, I also benefit from the ritual of confession—telling my sins to a priest and receiving through him the absolution of Christ. Christ told his Apostles, *"Whose sins you forgive are forgiven them. Whoever's sins you retain are retained."* (John 20:23). Many find this ritual strange. To me, the ritual has the beauty of something elegant and true.

For this ritual, I first consider my past deeds and faults since my last confession, whether of commission or omission, forming a firm purpose not to commit these sins again. I then enter the confessional, kneel and say, *"Bless me, Father, for I have sinned."* I recite the sins, explaining the circumstance as need be, and conclude, *"For these sins and all the sins I have forgotten, I am sorry."* The priest will usually offer some words of counsel, and he imposes a nominal penance—usually some small prayers. He then asks me to make an act of contrition. I use the formula I learned as a child. *"Oh my God, I am heartily sorry for having offended you, and I detest all my sins because I dread the loss of heaven and the pains of hell. But most of all, because they offend you, my God, who is all good, and worthy of all my love. I firmly resolve, with the help of your grace, to confess my sins, to do penance, and to amend my life. Amen."* The priest then speaks the words of absolution. *"God, the Father of mercies, through the death and resurrection of his son has reconciled the world to himself and poured out the Holy Spirit among us for the forgiveness of sins. Through the ministry of the Church may God grant you pardon and peace. And I absolve you from your sins in the name of the Father, and of the Son, and of the Holy Spirit."* I thank the priest and leave the confessional, offering my penance and some prayers for the priest before I leave the church.

When I know I have done wrong and find myself in need of Christ's mercy, I make time for this confession of my sins. It allows me to contemplate what is out of sync in my life and how to act the next time I face the same temptation. The oral confession of sins requires me to put into words what I did wrong, to be specific in acknowledging my guilt, and to move away from a generic *I guess I shouldn't have* to identifying my sins by name. The words externalize both my guilt and my acknowledgement of guilt. They help me mark the internal spirit of contrition by external conduct.

The priest's counsel stems from years of training and hearing more confessions in a month than I have made in my lifetime. The penance the priest imposes is not intended as a substitute for Christ's mercy. Rather, it is often deliberately light, to emphasize our reliance on Christ's sacrifice. It simply highlights our need to partake in Christ's suffering, in our own small way.

The words of contrition seem a little archaic, but to me they feel like a well-worn path I walk in the woods. I know each line and word so that every visit brings back the old emotions, renewed.

Then comes absolution. Speaking in the person of Christ, the priest says the words of mercy: *"I absolve you of your sins."* For those who believe, this is like hearing Christ say, *"My child, your sins are forgiven. Go, and sin no more."* (Cf. John 8:11).

This sacred ritual allows me a path through self-criticism. I know I have caused my daughter trauma. I know my frustration and selfishness has caused her pain. My oversight has left her with one physical scar already, and I cannot tell how many emotional scars. But the sacrament of confession builds within me a habit of self-reflection, acknowledging my mistakes, striving to act with greater virtue in the future, and uniting myself to the sufferings of a merciful Christ. And in this way, I live in mercy.

Lesson Five

Connect to Others
Building a Care Network

Joyce and I still call it the Small Room.

It sits in a renowned children's hospital, on the prenatal floor. Joyce was twenty-two weeks pregnant. We spent the day moving between tests, consultations, and evaluations. Then they brought us to the Small Room.

It was a tiny space for tiny thinking, with a specialist, a resident, a social worker, Joyce, and me. Six people, including Elizabeth in utero. There we heard Elizabeth's first prognosis. There the specialist told us we should terminate Elizabeth's life.

I remember particularly the isolation in that crowded room. The day before, my wife surprised me with a thirtieth birthday party at my brother's house. That seemed a distant memory. Joyce and I had many people to turn to for advice and comfort. But they were not with us in the Small Room. We were alone, with a doctor in a white coat telling us we should end the pregnancy now.

I could see Joyce needed my help. She was deaf to the doctor's words, deaf as the specialist told us Elizabeth would likely require a lifetime of institutional care, if she left the hospital. Joyce was deaf to everything after the news that our child had a large cavity in her brain, and it would never heal.

Joyce needed me to handle the conversation. I tried. But by law, I had no say in whether Elizabeth would live or die. Joyce alone had the legal right to make the decision. And so when I spoke, and Joyce did not, the doctor turned the conversation to Joyce alone, so my opposition would not impede Joyce's right to choose.

I was alone, cut out of my daughter's life, and Joyce was alone, cut off from me, even as she sat next to me, wanting my help.

We carried with us that sense of isolation after we left that Small Room. Despite the love of family and friends, their words could not console us, and the grief of others was more than we could bear. Already we were building an emotional wall between us and our child, preparing ourselves for the worst.

Then our local perinatologist asked us to come to his office. He was the first to detect Elizabeth's brain malformation, at the twenty-week ultrasound. He wanted to meet with us, now that we knew more.

There were no tests or procedures. We just talked. He spoke of the uncertainties of congenital brain malformations. They may lead to death, but the brain often finds a way to survive. He then spoke of his personal experience in raising a special needs child, a daughter who died as a toddler. His message was the first to resonate with us after Elizabeth's diagnosis. He told us of the hardships and the joys we would face. He spoke of his doubts, even years later, about the decisions he made for his daughter. He spoke of his loss and how much he misses his child. It was a message of hope and pain, joy and sadness. It was a message of a life really lived.

This doctor connected us to a bereavement nurse at the local hospital. She managed prenatal cases of children who would not leave the hospital. She helped to guide their families through the trauma of loss, in surroundings designed to celebrate new life. She told us we were not her ordinary patients, because Elizabeth might go home. She told us she would be with us to hear the story Elizabeth would tell. She knew how to climb walls and tear through ceilings in the hospital. With one call, she arranged a meeting with the director of the pediatric intensive care unit, to see if the local hospital could accommodate Elizabeth's delivery.

Slowly, slowly we turned the corner. Joyce decided to re-embrace the joy of pregnancy, come what may. Her friends hosted a shower, and when we went into the hospital six weeks early to deliver Elizabeth, good friends finished assembling her new furniture, leaving behind a large sign welcoming Elizabeth home.

Parenting a child with severe special needs isolates you. The trauma of the diagnosis creates barriers to relationships. Those who have not experienced the fear and grief cannot understand, or so it seems. Children in the community thrive as your child falls behind, and therapists insist more must be done. The difficulty others have in encountering your child, even as they engage ordinary children, may become an unspoken offense. The challenge of negotiating a world made for the able-bodied, or the fear of a public meltdown, persuades you not to go or do what you want. Staying at home, in a controlled environment, is so much easier. And for want of a qualified substitute caregiver, time away from your child may be impossible. These experiences shrink your world, until you cannot see beyond the caregiving obligations. Quietly, isolation becomes the norm.

Yet Scripture teaches us the importance of human connection. Isolation from others was the one *"not good"* of creation— *"It is not good for the man to be alone. I will make a helper suited to him."* (Gen. 2:18). Christ knew that connection, not isolation, was the path to God. He broke bread with social outcasts, like prostitutes and tax collectors. (Matt. 9:9-13). He healed lepers, whose disease kept them from temple worship. (E.g., Mark 1:40-45). He cared for the crippled beggars on the streets. (E.g., Matt. 9:1-8). He expelled demons that drove people away from their community. (E.g., Matt. 8:28-34). And at the Last Supper, Christ identified his disciples as his friends. (John 15:15).

Christ showed particular concern for parents' isolation. Two stories specifically highlight this.

The first, from the Gospel of Luke (7:11-17), speaks of the widow of Nain.

> *Soon afterward Jesus journeyed to a city called Nain, and his disciples and a large crowd accompanied him. As he drew near to the gate of the city, a man who had died was being carried out, the only son of his mother, and she was a widow. A large crowd from the city was with her.*
>
> *When the Lord saw her, he was moved with compassion for her and said to her, "Do not weep." He stepped forward and touched the coffin; at this the bearers halted, and he said, "Young man, I tell you, arise!" The dead man sat up and began to speak, and Jesus gave him to his mother.*

No one asked Christ to intervene. No one begged him to raise this young man. Jesus was simply *"moved with compassion."* Yet Christ's compassion was not for the man, but for his mother—a widow, who lost her only son. Christ felt compassion. He commanded the man to rise and *"gave him to his mother."*

The second story comes from the Gospel of John (19:25-27), our first-hand account of the Crucifixion.

> *Standing by the cross of Jesus were his mother and his mother's sister, Mary the wife of Clopas, and Mary of Magdala. When Jesus saw his mother and the disciple there whom he loved, he said to his mother, "Woman, behold, your son." Then he said to the disciple, "Behold, your mother." And from that hour the disciple took her into his home.*

Joseph's total absence from the Gospel during Christ's ministry suggests that Mary, the mother of Jesus, was a widow at this time. She is like the widow of Nain, watching her son die. Unwilling to reject his Father's plan, but still feeling compassion for his mother, Christ commits her to the care of his disciple, whom he loved. (John 21:20). John's own mother was still alive, and even watching the events from a distance. (Matt. 27:54-56). But even so, John accepted his sonship to Mary at Christ's request.

Christ appreciated our need to connect to others. We parents of special needs children must take this lesson to heart. We must connect to others.

The caregiving system is fragile when fewer people are integrated into a child's care. If the primary caregiver experiences a medical emergency, a substitute caregiver may not have the experience and knowledge to attend to the child. And isolation escalates not only the emotional costs of caregiving, but also the physical risks. Lifting and carrying Elizabeth takes a toll on my body. If I were the sole caregiver, I would have little opportunity to give my body rest. Moreover, involving more people improves the overall care. One caregiver will notice a new development the others overlooked, or they may independently confirm a change in the child's behaviors. One will remember something that worked in the past, or discover a better way of providing for the child's daily needs. Simply put, two minds—or three, or four—are better than one.

Joyce and I cope with the extraordinary childcare demands by a division of labor. Joyce manages the stream of paperwork that comes by mail. I handle prescriptions. Joyce covers local appointments that may pull her from work for an hour or two, while I cover appointments in Charlottesville at the University of Virginia.

We have developed a deep rapport with Elizabeth's pediatrician and regular specialists. My experience with medical experts in litigation helps me speak to them, and I learn all I can from them. During hospital stays in particular, I connect with the nursing staff. It makes the inherent frustrations more tolerable. You also learn how to work with the staff to care for your child. For Elizabeth, this means using music to calm her as they give her shots or shine lights in her eyes. It means speaking soft words to wake her before the nurse pokes and prods. It means warning the staff of the challenges they face, to avoid complications: low vision, tiny veins, an inability to understand spoken directions, and Elizabeth's propensity to put wires and tubes in her mouth.

Joyce and I decided early not to limit our family to Elizabeth merely because of her condition. We knew this would create challenges, but the children would learn care and compassion with Elizabeth, and Elizabeth would experience affection and love through siblings. Becky was born less

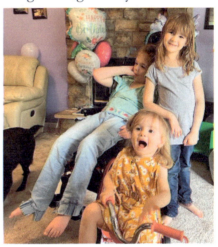

than nineteen months after Elizabeth. Marie came almost four years later. As I write this, we expect Philip to join his sisters within six weeks. Today, I covered the three girls at mass, as my pregnant wife rested at home. When I stepped away from the pew with Marie, Becky slid down next to Elizabeth and held her hand. When we got home, I poured some peanuts for Marie to enjoy. She carried one to Elizabeth and set it on her tongue. There is no substitute for the love of a sibling.

We employ a nanny as a joint caregiver, and the staff at school adds another line of support. Sharing information with so many caregivers can be difficult. If I cover an appointment and spend twenty minutes in a rapid-fire conversation with a specialist, I may not remember to communicate everything to my wife and nanny at home. But at least they know I know that doctor's perspective.

Both Joyce and I live far from our parents and siblings, but we know the place Elizabeth holds in their hearts. Aunt Carrie, for instance, has babysat her nieces during visits so Joyce and I can enjoy some time to ourselves. Uncle Greg and Aunt Chelle—Elizabeth's Godparents—have traveled the distance for birthdays and other special occasions, and even hosted a birthday celebration for Elizabeth. The Grandmas both take time to sing to Elizabeth, and they know all the best songs.

Our friends have made Elizabeth as much a part of their lives as our other children, or more. Several go out of their way to engage Elizabeth. We prefer to host our friends, as our house is more accessible for Elizabeth, but when we go to their house, they are quick to carry her wheelchair up stairways or to move baby gates that obstruct doorways. Someone will often step in to help her if Joyce and I step away.

Joyce and I have also joined a marriage ministry, gathering monthly with a small collection of families for dinner and discussion. Elizabeth stays with the adults, as the children play in the basement, because her limitations may be too much for a babysitter.

Joyce, during this pregnancy, cannot lift Elizabeth from her wheelchair into her bed. We rely on neighbors when Joyce and I have to go out in the evening, together or separately, and cannot take Elizabeth with us.

Our bosses and coworkers have proven extremely generous, not counting the cost of our time away. The question they ask tends to be, "Is there anything you need?"

We have also often experienced the kindness of strangers, going out of their way to hold doors or to help with the wheelchair at curbs. In Roanoke, far from home one weekend, Elizabeth's wheelchair broke. It was no longer safe to use. Joyce made some calls, and a volunteer at a local community center met us on a Saturday so we could borrow a secondhand wheelchair. Another time, I struck up a conversation with a woman painting in her art studio in Fredericksburg. As I told her Elizabeth's story, she suddenly grew excited. "I think I was praying for her before she was born!" she said. Elizabeth was on many prayer lists that winter, and many people will never know the fruit of their prayers.

One great blessing has been the chance to counsel others who are facing an adverse diagnosis with their child. I channel the wisdom of our perinatologist. "Tell me what's going on," I will say, to learn their child's condition and prognosis, their immediate concerns, and their needs. I sympathize with them, but I don't pity them or provide assurances that things will be alright. I tell them instead it will be difficult. I tell them it's a hell of a thing what they're going through, and they will need to be strong. I assure them that often there are no right answers, but merely the decisions you make with the information available. Then I try to give them the practical knowledge I have, such as how to get enrolled in Medicaid in Virginia.

Our church community has been particularly helpful. Joyce and I met through the parish, and it has watched our family grow. They know to expect Elizabeth kicking away at her wheelchair and clapping during the songs at the 8:30 a.m. Sunday mass.

At church, week after week, you watch others, and they watch you. We noticed the families with special needs children—those on autism spectrum or with Down's syndrome especially. Eventually we began to connect with the families, knowing we speak the same language and have some experiences in common. A few years ago, my wife and two other mothers launched a ministry called Special Blessings—a Catholic support group for the caregivers of those with special needs. We gather periodically for speakers and prayer, for socials and sharing.

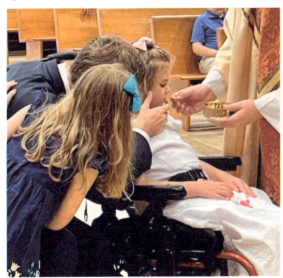

And today, our family celebrated a very special event. Through our parish, Elizabeth was among five special needs children to receive First Holy Communion—the highest connection with Christ any person might achieve on earth: intimate union with Jesus in his body, blood, soul, and divinity. I had the privilege of proclaiming the Old Testament reading at the mass. I tried not to choke up as I read about a bride bedecked with her jewels (Is. 61:9-11), looking down at Elizabeth in a beautiful white dress sown by her Grandmother.

Elizabeth sat in her chair, listening during the mass. When the time came, our pastor approached her with a small portion of the consecrated host. He touched it to her lips, and she opened her mouth and received it—Christ in the flesh.

> *"Amen, amen, I say to you, unless you eat the flesh of the Son of Man and drink his blood, you do not have life within you. Whoever eats my flesh and drinks my blood has eternal life, and I will raise him on the last day. For my flesh is true food, and my blood is true drink. Whoever eats my flesh and drinks my blood remains in me and I in him. Just as the living Father sent me and I have life because of the Father, so also the one who feeds on me will have life because of me. This is the bread that came down from heaven. Unlike your ancestors who ate and still died, whoever eats this bread will live forever."* (John 6:53-58).

The sacrament was all the more remarkable for two other events this week. Just three days ago, Elizabeth experienced severe seizures and vomiting. We were convinced her shunt failed again, and we prepared for another surgery. On the way to the hospital, I stopped by the church. I met one of the priests on his way to the confessional. I asked him to administer Last Rites, just in case the worst should happen. This is the sacrament of the sick—those who face some concrete risk of death. I wheeled Elizabeth from the van, and Father anointed her in the rain, in the parking lot of the church. Elizabeth stayed at the hospital two nights for observation and to adjust her medicine, and they released her the day before her First Communion.

And the morning they released Elizabeth, we learned the Supreme Court overturned *Roe v. Wade* and *Planned Parenthood v. Casey*, the decisions that declared a woman had a federal constitutional right to abort a child. *Planned Parenthood v. Casey*, in fact, was the case that said I had no right, in the Small Room, to oppose the termination of Elizabeth's life in utero, if Joyce chose. These decisions were overruled, allowing the states to regulate abortion.

The dissenting judges in that decision criticized the majority, saying, "[A]fter today's ruling, some States may compel women to carry to term a fetus with severe physical anomalies—for example, one afflicted with Tay-Sachs disease, sure to die within a few years of birth." This attitude promotes isolation of the worst sort. A child "sure to die within a few years of birth" is nothing, it seems, just because we hope to live three score years and ten. A child should die because she has special needs, rather than live a life—however long or short—with this condition, experiencing the world as her body allows. We should deprive her of the gift of connecting with others, because suffering with her is inconvenient.

As my daughter received communion today, I pondered the remarkable contrast between this day and the conversation in the Small Room:

In that Small Room, we were told there was no hope. Today, Elizabeth communed with God.

In the Small Room, we were isolated from family, friends, and spiritual counselors. Today, they surrounded us to join in this celebration.

In the Small Room, we were told Elizabeth had a broken brain, and her life wasn't worth the trouble of continuing the pregnancy. Some justices of the Supreme Court appear to agree. Today, she was a fitting temple for Christ to repose, in his body and soul.

In that Small Room, we were offered her death as a path to avoid suffering. Today, Elizabeth received the promise of life through union with Christ, who suffered, died, and rose from the grave.

In the Small Room we were isolated from all others, and from one another. Today, our daughter experienced the greatest connection of all—Jesus in the flesh, the Son of God.

.

Lesson Six

Sacrifice Is Joy
Loving Through the Suffering

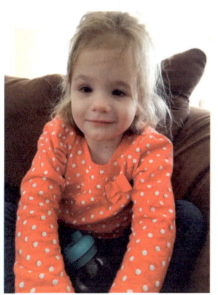

Elizabeth's "Ahhhh" calls me to her bedroom. "Good morning, Lizzie Belle," I say, before starting a song. *"Lizzie Belle, Lizzie Belle, oh hoh oh hoh hoh. Lizzie Bell. Bah-dat-dat-dah."* Elizabeth stops and listens.

I grab a diaper and heave open the wall of Elizabeth's bed. An Amish company crafted this beautiful wood bedframe as an alternative to the industrial medical models. The padded sides keep Elizabeth safe from falling.

Elizabeth notices I stopped singing and gives me a few "hnnns" from her throat as she wags her arms over her chest. I rest my hand gently on her. "Good morning, Elizabeth. It's Sunday. We have to go to church today." With both arms, I lift her onto her pillow, closer to me.

I start another song as I change her diaper. Ten thousand repetitions taught Elizabeth this process, and she does not resist. But the Botox in her leg muscles has nearly worn off, so they are stiff, nearly rigid, from her cerebral palsy. I gently press each knee until the muscle gives way, and the leg bends.

As I change the diaper, Becky plods down the stairs. I tell her we have church today and send her to the kitchen for breakfast. She will have cereal with a side of bacon. Marie calls from upstairs, so after securing Elizabeth's fresh diaper, I close the bed, turn on the radio, and give my youngest daughter a piggy-back ride down the stairs.

With Marie strapped into her booster seat near Becky, munching on cereal and bacon, I return to Elizabeth. Opening the drawers under the bed, I pick an outfit. Elizabeth never has enough clothes. She goes through them so quickly with spills and smears and leaks. The day promises to be hot, but large air conditioning vents lie next to the handicap seating we use at the church, so I find a light shirt with long sleeves.

I sit Elizabeth on the edge of the bed as I change her clothes. A glance around me shows her wheelchair is not at hand, but no matter. I step to Elizabeth's right. With one arm across her back and another arm under her legs, I sweep her from the bed and set her right hip against mine. This is easier when she is a little rigid—one way we rely on an adverse medical condition in our routine. She is now a little more than seventy pounds, down almost fifteen pounds since we switched her medications.

I carry her to the door, down the hallway, and into the living room. Her wheelchair is not positioned well, so I put Elizabeth in her recliner, and raise the footrest so she won't slide off. I ask Becky if she has seen the TV remote, and she gives me some vague, mostly imagined help. I find it on the couch. Turning on the music app, I decline Becky's request for the "funny station" but compromise with showtunes. Elizabeth smiles and shakes her arms excitedly as she hears the opening song of a popular movie musical.

Joyce is upstairs, beginning the transformation from looking beautiful to looking beautiful for the public. I assemble her breakfast, the task interrupted when Elizabeth called me. I plate green grapes next to the now-lukewarm eggs and room-temperature bacon, hoping the natural sugars and protein will help Joyce to make it through mass. Her pregnancy with Philip continues to take a toll. I deliver the food to the hers-and-hers sink in our bedroom, for Joyce to find after she showers.

Downstairs, Elizabeth is kicking and rocking to a song she knows. Becky asks if she can be done with breakfast, and Marie tries to copy her. "All done," Marie says in a two-year old's mostly intelligible English. I send Becky to change her clothes and find her shoes as I release Marie from the booster seat.

Elizabeth's breakfast goes with mine on a single plate, and I count out Elizabeth's medicine. She gets six pills in the morning now, down from nine pills. I use one fork for our joint breakfast. Two forks inevitably get crossed, and keeping our germs apart is a fool's errand. Besides, incubating her germs in my body has helped me to know what she feels when she gets sick, so I can help her.

I plant a tiny pill on a forkful of eggs. The most important pills always go first. But Elizabeth doesn't want eggs. When I bring the fork to her mouth, she keeps her lips pressed shut. I try again and she twists her head away, putting an arm over her mouth, elbow out, communicating clearly, "Stop annoying me." I switch tactics. I wrap a pill with bacon and brush it against Elizabeth's cheek. This offering she finds acceptable. She drops her elbow and opens her mouth to receive it. Next comes a grape with a pill pressed inside. This, too, she accepts. Four pills to go. A few bites later, she shows her talent for cheeking pills. I foil her plan with a piece of fruit delivered to that side of her mouth.

After the pills and a bite or two more, I offer her the eggs once again. She squeezes her mouth shut. I don't know how she figures out my offerings so quickly, but she does, and she has strong opinions day to day.

Realizing she must be thirsty after the bacon, I search for a cup. Elizabeth can drink from an ordinary cup, but she will test its limits with her teeth and hands, and usually overturns it after a sip or two. On a Sunday, before mass, I assemble a sippy cup instead.

Shouting from Becky and Marie interrupts me. Becky has a toy Marie wants. At a glance, I have to decide whether to say "Share" or "Don't take." But I see another option. "Becky, I told you to get your shoes on. Marie, go find your shoes." I hear protests, but I hold the line.

Elizabeth has become pickier about what she will drink. Warm white milk or cold chocolate milk used to be reliable, but not anymore. Water is hit and miss. We don't keep juice in the house. Inspiration strikes. I pour some of my morning tea into the sippy cup, add her daily laxative powder, and an ice cube. Elizabeth accepts it and starts drinking.

The hour has been slipping away, and I still need to change Marie, get shoes on two girls, and find my own shoes. Five days a week my wife or nanny gets the girls ready, and Joyce and I cooperate on Saturdays, but Sunday mornings are mine. I snatch Marie and playfully charge up the stairs, to find her an outfit. After putting it on Marie, I stop by my bedroom to check for my shoes and check my wife's status, before giving Marie another piggy-back ride down the stairs.

We are short on time, as always, but I try to get Elizabeth a few more bites. She generally tells me how hungry she is by how quickly and widely she opens her mouth when food is near. She is not interested. I pull the wheelchair close and lift her into it. It's time for shoes.

Marie struts around with a smile, proud she has one shoe. Of course, that means the other could be anywhere. I search as Joyce comes downstairs. She turns Elizabeth's music down. She seems to think the music is too loud, simply because the music is too loud. I spot Marie's shoe in the dining room, with the sock still stuck inside, and ask Joyce if she has seen my shoes. She has, because they are in plain sight. I put Marie in my lap and pull her socks and shoes on her, put my own on, and turn back to Elizabeth.

Elizabeth wears ankle-foot orthotic braces—AFOs—to stretch her Achilles tendon. To assemble this footwear, I start with knee-length socks. Then each AFO comes in two parts—a molded foot piece sitting inside a shell that extends up her calf. Finally, I grab the extra-wide specialty shoes, with a zipper that opens the entire top. Socks, AFOs, and shoes. Eight foot pieces so she can ride in her wheelchair in public.

Joyce has already ushered the two younger girls to the van, because we are nearly late. I guide the wheelchair to the front door, as the door into the

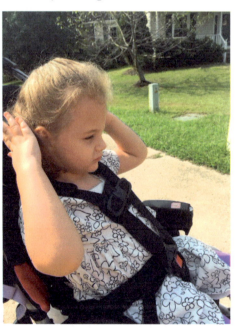

garage cannot accommodate a ramp. I prop open the screen. It takes nearly every inch of space on the homemade platform outside the threshold to swing Elizabeth's wheelchair ninety degrees to the right, onto the plywood ramp down to the porch. Joyce struggles with Elizabeth on this ramp, but I have not jerry-rigged a better option. I roll Elizabeth to the porch's far end, then left onto a wooden platform, and then left again onto a long aluminum ramp. The ramp was a gift after an elderly man passed away. Like so many things in our lives with Elizabeth, it came exactly when we needed it.

We turn left toward the garage and our rear-loading, wheelchair-accessible minivan. It cost ten thousand dollars above the market price of the non-accessible vehicle, but we needed it. I lift the rear door and release the ramp, which folds out easily. I wheel Elizabeth in, trying to avoid the belts and toys and crackers that always clutter the path. I stop Elizabeth between her two sisters in their narrow jump seats, and start assembling Elizabeth's seatbelts. A waist belt and a four-point harness already bind Elizabeth to her chair. I lock the chair's brakes. Kneeling in the back of the van, I hook the chair with two anchors and snap a long seatbelt into place. Then I hook on one or two front anchors. Two seatbelts, a four-point harness, wheel breaks, and three to four anchors, all to keep Elizabeth safe in her wheelchair on a short drive.

As Joyce drives, Elizabeth begins vocalizing again. I sort through the possibilities. Those are not her happy sounds, but it is not severe pain. Boredom? No. It's discomfort. Hunger? Thirst? No. It may be constipation. I can't fix it, but I turn the radio to the classical station and give her a toy to distract her.

We arrive at church fifteen minutes later. We park in the handicap spot behind the building. Joyce retrieves Marie, and Becky scrambles out by herself. I get Elizabeth. Open the rear door and lower the ramp. Unbuckle the large seatbelt. Remove one, two, three anchors, maybe four. Release the wheel break. Back out of the van, avoiding the belts, toys, and crackers. Proceed to church.

Joyce falls behind as Marie dawdles. Becky and I walk with Elizabeth. A parishioner just ahead holds the heavy door for us, and I thank him. The ushers greet us. "Aren't you missing some people?" one jokes. "They're coming," I assure him. We take worship sheets and push on.

The semicircle of pews have several spaces for wheelchairs. None are ideal, but the best lie on the far left, in the second or third row. These are close enough to the front so my two girls can see, but they keep the wheelchair out of the communion line. We avoid the front row, though. We need the younger girls confined.

I sit next to Elizabeth. As the others open their missals, I lean toward Elizabeth and say a prayer, as she listens.

Some, looking from the outside, see the challenges of raising a special needs child. They see the hospital visits and the meltdowns, the public outburst and the physical limitations. *This is a tragedy*, they say. Others see the child's innocence and glory in it, overlooking the family's anxiety and stress. *The child is a little angel*, they say. Both are wrong. Raising the child is far different than they imagine.

Most days are routine. They may not be easy, but they are routine. Most days, God willing, don't involve hospitals. They involve a heightened form of childcare. The sacrifice is there. You still feel the weight of carrying your child. But it is the same sacrifice you experienced yesterday, and the day before. You know what it is like. You have done it before, and you can do it again.

But most tasks also involve intimacy, when you and your child each live in the space of your overlapping personalities. You each know the give and take of communicating without words, of compromising, of gently getting your way, of being there with and for the other.

The sacrifice and the intimacy are seamlessly entwined. Carrying your child, feeding your child, preparing her for the day, and living the day all involve moments of inseparable sacrifice and intimacy. The weight of my child as I walk down the hall gives me a sense of closeness, for very few occupy a place in this world where they can aid Elizabeth in this way. She depends on me. And I will make good on that trust.

Most days are routine. But not all days. Some days—some moments—call for great sacrifice. I recall Elizabeth's first surgery, installing the shunt. Her head ballooned from the fiftieth percentile at birth to above the ninety-fifth percentile five weeks later. The pediatrician dispatched us to UVA hospital—our first of countless visits. The hospital admitted Elizabeth, expecting to do the surgery in the morning. Elizabeth could not have any formula or breast milk after midnight.

The night was dreadful. Joyce was beyond exhausted. Elizabeth was hungry. A mother cannot listen to a five-week-old daughter cry with hunger. But the hospital would not do the surgery if Elizabeth had eaten. Sometime after midnight, I took Elizabeth into the hall and began to walk. Past the patient rooms. Past the nurses' desk. To the door of the unit. I then turned around and walked again. And again. And again. Trying to give Elizabeth comfort. Trying to keep her asleep. Letting my wife sleep in the room. Just walking, walking, walking, walking, walking. I whispered songs to Elizabeth when she stirred. Walking, walking. Past two o'clock. Past three o'clock and four. Walking. About six o'clock I found a chair outside the room. Elizabeth slept in my lap. I tried to rest without nodding off. The doctors started to come by. Joyce woke and took Elizabeth. The night had passed.

Sacrifice is a habit and a skill. We get better with practice. We learn better techniques. We learn our capacities lie beyond our expected limits. Discomfort becomes easier to tolerate. The moments of great sacrifice make the little sacrifices routine. And the little moments of intimacy prepare us for the challenges of great sacrifices. You reach the point when there is no doubt, no hesitancy, in accepting a sacrifice.

I sometimes hear, in religious circles, that if we are anxious, worried, or suffering, we are focused too much on the things of this world. We must turn our minds and our hearts back to Christ. Taken to the extreme, it says if we are suffering, we are not praying enough; we are too self-centered; we are doing something wrong. This Gospel of Wellbeing is not the Gospel of Christ. What does Paul say? *"A thorn in the flesh was given to me, an angel of Satan, to beat me, to keep me from being too elated. Three times I begged the Lord about this, that it might leave me, but he said to me, 'My grace is sufficient for you, for power is made perfect in weakness.'"* (2 Cor. 12:7-9). Paul, of all people, was no spiritual wimp. He was not distracted by the things of this world. And still he suffered. What is more, he prayed for relief from suffering, and Christ refused. The Lord says, *"My grace is sufficient for you."* The grace was finding purpose or meaning in the suffering, and being able to bear it, not taking it away.

Prayer will not expel suffering from our lives. On the contrary, *"Whom the Lord loves, he disciplines; he scourges every son he acknowledges."* (Heb. 12:6). The New Testament teaches us, at every turn, to embrace suffering. *"We even boast of our afflictions, knowing that affliction produces endurance, and endurance, proven character, and proven character, hope, and hope does not disappoint, because the love of God has been poured out into our hearts through the holy Spirit that has been given to us."* (Rom. 5:3-5). *"I rejoice in my sufferings for your sake, and in my flesh I do my share on behalf of His body, which is the church, in filling up what is lacking in Christ's afflictions."* (Col. 1:24).

"I rejoice in my sufferings." We should find joy in our sufferings. How is this possible? *"I rejoice in my sufferings for your sake."* We can find joy in suffering when it serves a purpose, when it is for the sake of something you love, or especially someone you love. Love allows you to imagine with emotional clarity the fruits of your sacrifice.

"[I]n my flesh I do my share on behalf of His body, which is the church, in filling up what is lacking in Christ's afflictions." What do Christ's afflictions lack? My presence, my participation. I cannot be present at the Cross of Christ in the same way that the Blessed Mother or St. John were present. I cannot stare at the suffering Christ, and be with him in his agony, as Mary and the beloved disciple were. But when I suffer for another, I experience some small part of what it was like to be there, when a grieving mother and bereft friend looked upon the man as he labored and died, knowing that they were doing all they could to console him, and knowing he knew they would do more if they could. Think of the pain they all felt—one directly, and the other two through love. Think of how they wished to spare each other the pain, but the relationship—being present to one another—was more important than avoiding pain.

The sacrifice changes you. You learn your limits are far beyond what you imagined in your fear. And with new confidence, you stand ready to embrace righteous suffering for the sake of you beloved one, you learn you are not in control, and you learn to trust in a generous God. *"[A]ffliction produces endurance, and endurance, proven character, and proven character, hope, and hope does not disappoint."*

As Joyce and I prepared to wed, our priest agreed to incorporate into his homily a reflection often used in nuptial masses before the 1970s.

My dear friends: You are about to enter upon a union which is most sacred and most serious. It is most sacred, because it is established by God himself, and most serious, because it will bind you together for life in a relationship so close and so intimate, that it will profoundly influence your whole future. That future, with its hopes and disappointments, its successes and its failures, its pleasures and its pains, its joys and its sorrows, is hidden from your eyes. You know that these elements are mingled in every life, and are to be expected in your own. And so not knowing what is before you, you take each other for better or for worse, for richer or for poorer, in sickness and in health, until death. Truly, then, these words are most serious.

It is a beautiful tribute to your undoubted faith in each other, that recognizing their full import, you are, nevertheless, so willing and ready to pronounce them. And because these words involve such solemn obligations, it is most fitting that you rest the security of your wedded life upon the great principle of self-sacrifice. And so you begin your married life by the voluntary and complete surrender of your individual lives in the interest of that deeper and wider life which you are to have in common.

Henceforth you will belong entirely to each other; you will be one in mind, one in heart, and one in affections. And whatever sacrifices you may hereafter be required to make to preserve this mutual life, always make them generously. Sacrifice is usually difficult and irksome. Only love can make it easy, and perfect love can make it a joy. We are willing to give in proportion as we love. And when love is perfect, the sacrifice is complete.

God so loved the world that he gave his only-begotten Son, and the Son so loved us that he gave himself for our salvation. "Greater love than this no man hath, that a man lay down his life for his friends." (John 15:13). No greater blessing can come to your married life than pure conjugal love, loyal and true to the end. May, then, this love with which you join your hands and hearts today never fail, but grow deeper and stronger as the years go on. And if true love and the unselfish spirit of perfect sacrifice guide your every action, you can expect the greatest measure of earthly happiness that may be allotted to man in this vale of tears. The rest is in the hands of God.

Nor will God be wanting to your needs. He will pledge you the life-long support of his graces in the Holy Sacrament which you are now going to receive.

As we heard these words from the priest, Joyce and I expected to have children. We expected to learn the ordinary challenges of married life and parenting. We had no reason to expect we would parent a special needs child. Now, years later, I bless God that we heard these words on our wedding day, for they mean more to me now than I ever imagined they could.

Love can make sacrifice easy, and perfect love can make it a joy. I have not lived up to the calling of perfect love. Too often I have been short tempered or prone to frustration. But I have seen enough to know this line is true. Love can make sacrifice easy, and perfect love can make it a joy.

As I sit at Elizabeth's feet in the evening, caressing the creases on her skin from a day of wearing her AFOs, I marvel at her fortitude. I marvel at my privilege to be there at this moment, offering her this gentle relief. I think of Christ washing the feet of his disciples, as a sign of their duty to serve. When I carry Elizabeth to and from her bed, I feel her seventy pounds heavy on my arms, and I think what a blessing it is that I have been given my arms and legs and muscles for this purpose. She is a heavy load, but not as heavy as the Cross. *"Whoever wishes to come after me must deny himself, and take up his cross, and follow me."* (Matt. 16:24). *"Take my yoke upon you and learn from me, for I am meek and humble in heart; and you will find rest for yourselves. For my yoke is easy and my burden is light."* (Matt. 11:29-30).

Elizabeth has a far, far more beautiful soul than I will ever have. She takes the suffering so often without a sign of protest. And if, through my body, she gets to live, then my body is well used. My hand holds the fork that feeds her. My voice turns her expressions into words. My arms hold her and my legs walk for her. The brain that manages her body is broken, and so I offer her my brain and body. I get to be there for her, to allow her to encounter something beyond her own natural limits. And through this, she has carried me far beyond the limits I assumed I had.

I rejoice in my sufferings. I experience the sacrifice with joy. In my flesh I do some small part in filling up what is lacking in Christ's afflictions. Through my sacrifice, I aid and console Elizabeth, as Mary and John consoled the crucified Christ by their presence. Sacrifice is joy.

LOVE FIERCELY

Accept the Preparation
Seeing God in Your Story

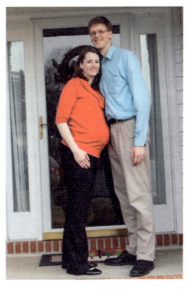

God works in ordinary ways—most of the time. Like a playwright, he usually avoids being seen, but his creative hand shapes every inch of the world we know. Still, now and then, he offers a glimpse of his presence: in a sticky coincidence, or in deep faith unreasonably rewarded, or the unremitting whisper of things to come. And through these gentle impressions, he guides and prepares us to be the people we will be called to be, in a play that spans countless generations.

We parents of special needs children may find great comfort when we see in our lives God's role in preparing us for this vocation, or signs that he is with us on this journey. We must lean into those experiences, recognizing them as graces given to us for consolation and solace.

Joyce and I both come from families that experienced the loss of a child. My mother delivered her oldest daughter prematurely, on my mother's birthday, and the little girl died the next day. Though I never met her, we grew up remembering my sister in our nighttime prayers. "Good night, Jennifer," we'd say. "Keep us out of mischief." Joyce likewise had an older brother who passed away, from a rare form of cancer, when she was seven and he was fourteen. Losing a child was more than just an imagined possibility for us.

From kindergarten through twelfth grade, I attended a non-diocesan Catholic school operated by families in the community. Grades came easy, and I filled my time with extracurriculars. In my junior year, we formed a pro-life club, adopting the motto "All human life is precious—born and unborn." We educated ourselves, engaged in advocacy, and periodically prayed at an abortion facility. In my senior year, I became the club president. Then I attended a small Catholic college, Christendom, in Front Royal, Virginia. I maximized my class load and minimized my study time, pouring myself into extracurriculars. I joined the college pro-life group, which prayed and counseled at an abortion facility in Washington, D.C. every Saturday.

Each week, the abortion facilities scheduled volunteers to escort its patrons past our peaceful, praying students and around our counselors, into the facility. I sometimes surprised my colleagues with the comment that the escorts were very much like us. We both sacrificed Saturday mornings to be on this street, on opposite sides of the issue. But for the grace of God, there go I. By senior year, I became the president of the pro-life group.

I came to accept a creed of sincere reliance on God. My intellectual powers depended on God's inspiration. If I did good work now for God through my extracurriculars, God's Spirit would be with me in my moment of need. I could pour hours into an uninspired paper and produce uninspired results. Or I could pray with the pro-life group in the morning and rest on God's inspiration in the afternoon. Many times I found myself on a Saturday evening discarding half of a half-decent paper due Monday, stirred by an exceptional idea. I took the law school admissions exam, looking at the thick study guides only the evening before the test, and then getting a good night's sleep. It was not arrogance, but faith. My time was better spent on projects for the community.

On faith I applied to only one law school—Ave Maria School of Law— and it offered me a handsome scholarship. In law school, I joined the pro-life group, and after my first semester, I was elected president for a year. God blessed me, allowing me good grades while also developing strong professional credentials. By my final year, I had the sense that I didn't need to see my next step in life. My task was to pick my foot up and put it down, while God would lay out the road ahead of me.

I entered the legal market in a terrible economy, after the 2008 financial collapse. Scarce job interviews produced no offers, until I got a call from Fredericksburg. A non-lawyer wanted to organize a network of professional firms. He wanted me to establish a law firm. In a rash move, I accepted.

The day I moved to Fredericksburg, at a store, I ran into a friend from the law school pro-life group. She invited me to a new young adult group at the local parish. Three months later, bowling with the young adults, I met Joyce. We exchanged emails about *Pride and Prejudice*, and I asked her on a date. While, in the next year, we each considered moving away from Fredericksburg, she applied to a new job within her company, and I applied to a litigation firm in Richmond, based on a Craigslist posting. Within days of each other, we learned we each got our job. Nine months later, we were engaged.

God had blessed me abundantly. He guided me down extraordinary paths, gently, gently all the time. But I sensed something new. In the Gospels, Peter professes his faith in Christ's divinity, and Christ promptly tries to prepare his disciples for the Crucifixion. (Matt. 6:13-23). Similarly, I felt an unreasoned confidence God was preparing me for a great challenge. A challenge so severe it could break me.

This premonition grew within me, and I told Joyce. My sincerity frightened her a little. But God continued to bless us. We found a house in the perfect neighborhood; Joyce was promoted; and I closed a case unexpectedly, allowing us to pay off the wedding by the day we married.

Then came the miscarriage, about six months after our wedding. The doctor at the eight-week appointment found a blighted ovum—an empty shell in place of an embryo. Weeks later, when the miscarriage finally occurred, the bleeding became so bad I took Joyce to the emergency room. By the next morning, Joyce was in surgery, as I wandered the halls anxiously. Sometime later, Joyce found herself holding another positive pregnancy test, but she miscarried again within weeks.

Joyce asked me soon after if I thought the miscarriages were the challenge we would face. They had been hard, but I told her I did not think so. I still heard the whisper of a coming crisis. The miscarriages felt like preparation.

We were cautious when Joyce became pregnant a third time. She made it through the first few weeks, and then the first appointment. But morning sickness came with a fury, unremitting and uncontrolled, night and day. Once or twice a week, Joyce required IV fluids, unable to keep hydrated. She received an intravenous PICC line for antinausea medication and fluids. One morning, our dog tangled herself in the tubing and pulled the PICC line out of Joyce's arm, putting us back in the emergency room. Another line became infected and had to be replaced. But slowly, slowly, she turned the corner. Nineteen weeks into the pregnancy, Joyce had the PICC line removed.

A perinatologist covered the twenty-week ultrasound. His technician thoroughly scanned our child's anatomy, measuring bones and organs. She told us we were having a girl. We knew Elizabeth would be her name, a call back to our *Pride and Prejudice* discussions.

I remember my joy. It had been a long pregnancy already, and a long journey before. And now we knew it was for a little girl we would name Elizabeth.

The perinatologist came in. He was calm and personable. He took time to ask us our names and about the pregnancy, and then he gently told us the news. They could see something was wrong. Elizabeth's brain was not formed right. The doctor raised the option of abortion, but he accepted our decision when we declined. We needed to get more people involved. He arranged for us to be seen at a nationally renowned children's hospital.

At home, I called my mother to share the news. It was her birthday. We were both thinking of Jennifer, my mother's oldest daughter, who would have been celebrating her own birthday. I am sure Joyce's family thought of her brother.

Two weeks later, we sat across from a doctor in the Small Room, after hours of tests and consultations. The doctor asked our baby's name. We said Elizabeth. The doctor explained that imaging showed a gaping cavity in Elizabeth's brain. She conscientiously referred to Elizabeth by her name. She told us the brain malformation could not be fixed, and the condition would likely progress in utero. She told us Elizabeth would not likely survive to term, or if she did, she would not leave the hospital, or if she did, she would require a lifetime of institutional care.

Joyce was overwhelmed, and I knew where the conversation was going. The doctor would recommend abortion. She would look to Joyce for an answer. I knew I had no legal say in the decision. I asked questions about the diagnosis and prognosis, but hesitated to broach the topic we had to discuss.

Joyce did not see this. To Joyce, doctors cure and treat, and abortion is not healthcare, no matter the child's condition. And so she told the doctor we would probably do whatever the doctor recommends.

Not once did the doctor use the word abortion. She may have talked of termination—I don't remember. But that was the message. She told us they would arrange for the deliberate death of Elizabeth, my daughter, even while using her name! They had to act quickly. State law allowed the procedure only in the next two weeks, since Joyce's life was not in real jeopardy. They would arrange for it within days.

I knew Joyce could not respond. I knew she wanted me to take the lead. I knew it was a fool's errand, but I had to try for my wife's sake. I wanted to be gentle, to turn the discussion to other options, without becoming emotional. I told the doctor, with a fragile voice, that we were Catholic, and we did not believe in abortion. That was not a problem, she assured us. They do this procedure for people of all faiths in these circumstances: Christians, Muslims, Jews.

I tried more directly to steer the conversation toward other options. The doctor could sense my resistance but refused to cooperate. She turned her attention exclusively to Joyce, who was not in a frame of mind to give informed consent.

What scared me most was not my powerlessness. It was not my honest fear that this deliberate pressure might overcome Joyce's resistance. What scared me was that abortion made sense. *Why not reset this pregnancy? Why not let Elizabeth go, if she would have a lifetime of pain and never make it out of medical institutions? Why not?*

Why not?

But *I* was pro-life. Back in law school, I would tell my friend every day, "Ain't life great." As the classes grew difficult, my friend expressed half-sincere skepticism. He could accept life was worth living, he said, because Bishop Fulton Sheen said that, and he could trust Bishop Sheen. But he wanted me to prove life was great. I showed him that my hero, Pope John Paul II, said life was truly a good. My friend nodded and agreed, and said he could trust the late Polish Pope. But soon he pointed out that *good* was not *great*. I told him I would prove to him that life was great. I didn't know how, but I would prove it to his satisfaction. In a few moments I had it. Pope John Paul II's encyclical *Evangelium Vitae* proclaims, *"Truly great must be the value of human life if the Son of God has taken it up and made it the instrument of the salvation of all humanity!"* My friend laughed and agreed with me. Life was great.

How could I, after all my pro-life work, consider abortion as an option? I couldn't. *I* couldn't. Abortion made sense, but it was wholly unacceptable. I couldn't choose abortion. Still, it scared me that abortion made sense. *But for the grace of God.* But for the grace of God.

Science shows we are not good at making decisions in the face of bad news about the future. An adverse diagnosis for our child in utero disrupts our hopes and plans, replacing them with uncertainty and fear. We focus on pain and suffering, and what will change for the worse, not the things in life that will remain the same or improve. We undervalue and underestimate our coping skills. We cannot foresee how we will adapt to the new reality. And so, we overestimate both how bad we will feel and how long we will feel bad, and choose abortion to avoid the experience.

Families in these situations want a child—a healthy child—not an abortion. The stories of these mothers, recorded in medical literature, wrench the heart. Often they must begin the abortion by taking a pill at home. But this makes them an active participant, not simply someone that allowed the process to happen. They struggle with that deliberate act, staring at the pill, reluctant to participate. Later, they don't want to tell themselves or others that they had an abortion, but instead want their child's life to be acknowledged. They prefer the narrative that they lost the child because of the health condition, not that they elected an abortion.

Doctors delivering the bad news must discuss the option of a legal abortion and must decide how to frame the discussion. Doctors who expect the family to choose abortion will often emphasize worse-case scenarios and use language like "low quality of life." This usually reduces the stress and the regret associated with abortion. A physician experienced in these conversations knows to acknowledge the pregnancy, and may therefore use the child's name.

But for those inclined to reject an abortion, this increases the trauma, and it may contribute to serious psychological struggles following the abortion. One study showed that four months after terminating a pregnancy because of an adverse prenatal diagnosis, almost half of the women were experiencing post-traumatic stress and more than a quarter were experiencing depression. Those most likely to resist an abortion for religious, age, or other reasons are most likely to suffer severe psychological consequences if they surrender to the pressure. But if the family moves forward with the pregnancy, another study shows the emotional distress returns to almost normal levels by delivery.

These conversations don't need to follow that script. The doctor should not default to worst-case scenarios. Shocking bad news may overwhelm the parents. Since the parents tend to dwell on the child's pain or disabilities, the medical staff should help the family to see the positive experiences that child may have. The physician can help the parents recall how they coped and adapted to challenging circumstances before. The doctor should look for signs the family opposes abortion, and disclose the risks of post-traumatic stress and depression. Informed consent requires these disclosures. And the parents should not be pressed for an immediate decision, as it takes time to adjust to the new reality.

But the doctor may not be a neutral advisor. She will have a general opinion about abortion, and she will likely have an opinion about abortion in this case. She may fear being sued if the family decides against an abortion and later regrets it. She can safely present a worse-case scenario, because the few who decline the abortion will assume they simply beat the odds—that their child is a miracle baby. And the doctor may not have time to allow for grief, if the window for a legal abortion will soon close. The doctor may need a prompt decision, and the doctor might frame the conversation so as to get it.

But Joyce and I did not know this in that lonely, Small Room. The doctor pressed Joyce for a decision—for *the decision*—but the doctor did not get it. After an eternity, someone suggested we may need a few minutes alone. Joyce shattered the moment they left. She embraced me, crying out her pain, crying out her disappointment and frustration. She did not want to see the doctor again. Joyce did not want to look at the woman who could speak Elizabeth's name as she told us to end our daughter's life.

I suppressed my grief as well as I could. I tried to brace my wife to face the doctors and give them our decision, so we could get out of this pathetic room. We called the doctor back in. I told them we would go forward with the pregnancy, and Joyce nodded her affirmation.

Driving home, Joyce asked me what I thought. I told my wife that I hoped my child died. I thought of my sister, Jennifer. I cried as I said, in broken words, that I would rather have a daughter in heaven than struggling in a hospital surrounded by machines and medical staff.

This crisis brought me close to the brink, close to doing something that would leave me unable to forgive myself. But God prepared me. He gave me a loving family, and the memory of a sister I never knew. Inch by inch, he cultivated my capacity to trust in him. He allowed me to grow into a man stubborn in my pro-life identity, so that I could say *yes* to life even when my mind asked *"Why?"* He gave me the love of a strong woman who chose motherhood against medical advice, and at great cost. He gave us challenges to grow our strength to face adversity.

It took months for us to reengage the joy of pregnancy, but one day out of the blue, Joyce told me she was going to stop acting as though things would turn out for the worst, and she was going to expect them to be all right in the end.

Morning sickness continued to dog Joyce, though she managed it with medication. She kept her upbeat outlook even as early signs of preeclampsia appeared.

Preeclampsia is the preliminary signs of a dangerous condition. It progresses to eclampsia, and can lead to death. It is cured only by delivery before the symptoms go too far.

Now our doctors had to decide when to induce delivery, to end the preeclampsia, while trying to prolong the pregnancy to allow Elizabeth's lungs to develop. Meanwhile, Elizabeth's head was continuing to swell because of the hydrocephalus. If it swelled too much, they would need to perform a caesarean section. But if the preeclampsia progressed too far, it could preclude this, because Joyce would lose platelets and her blood may not clot after the surgery.

Joyce and I discussed what to do if we had to choose between Joyce and Elizabeth, and how much risk to accept to both before we made that call. Abortion was not an option, but we may have to choose who would bear the risks. For Joyce, there was no debate: *Save Elizabeth*. But if the choice fell to me, I don't know what I would have done.

Six weeks before the due date, the doctor called Joyce. A test showed the preeclampsia advancing quickly. She was admitted and monitored closely. She received steroids to strengthen Elizabeth's lungs. As the days progressed, Joyce's platelet count dropped precipitously low. Surgical delivery was impossible and even an epidural was too dangerous. Joyce had to choose between vaginal delivery under general anesthesia, or delivery with only short-duration pain medications. She chose to be awake.

Many people prayed for us throughout the pregnancy, and many were praying for us that week. My sister is in Mother Theresa's order, the Missionaries of Charity. I have another sister in the Nashville Dominicans. From around the globe, prayers climbed to the heavens.

A week after Joyce's admission, the perinatologist told us they would either induce delivery that evening, or send her home for the weekend. An anxious, nervous excitement carried me away. Joyce, instead, painted her toenails.

At six-thirty that evening, a doctor broke Joyce's water. We watched television for a few hours as the pain increased. I tried to distract Joyce and help her along, but a husband will never score above a D+ in the labor and delivery room. I was no exception.

Joyce received one shot of pain medication. It lasted about fifteen minutes, and she hated how it made her feel. By two in the morning, she was in full labor, with the nurse coaching her. By two-thirty, the doctor was there. I was a nervous wreck, less helpful than a bowl of quivering fruit gelatin. Joyce was learning quickly how to bring a child into this world.

At 3:05 a.m., Joyce delivered Elizabeth. There she was, my beautiful, beautiful girl. She cried aloud as the nurse placed her in her mother's arms, a wonderful sound, a wonderful sight. The nursing team moved quickly, though, to get Elizabeth under the lights and check her vitals. She was strong, and despite everything, she appeared full of vigor and life.

The nursing team soon prepared to take Elizabeth to the NICU. I looked back to Joyce. "Go with her," she said, and I did.

I hope I will never forget that night, sitting with my daughter, in the corner of the NICU. I could feel my brain rewiring itself, to move from being a husband and man to being a father. The doctors could not imagine that Elizabeth was five weeks early, or that she faced serious health risks.

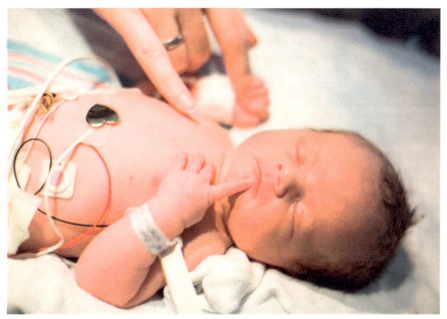

Joyce came in a wheelchair to see her little girl. We were a family, together in this way for the first time. My wife was still weak from the labor, especially with her low platelets, and she had to go back to the room. But there I sat, and watched, and marveled, and loved. It was February 14, St. Valentine's Day.

Two days later, in the presence of Joyce's mother and my brother, a priest came to the hospital and baptized Elizabeth. The next day, I brought Elizabeth home.

Since that day, I have not heard the silent word of God preparing me for a challenge to come, not like I did before. I have not felt the same confidence that I can walk into tomorrow without seeing the ground before me, the confidence that God will create my path. My confidence in God has not failed, but the feeling he gave me was a grace for the moment, the aid I needed at the time. Now I can trust in God because of a promise fulfilled.

He prepared me for this task. From the memory of my oldest sister lost hours after her birth, to the hours spent in pro-life prayer at abortion facilities, to the many opportunities to grow my faith in him, he has prepared me for this.

And although I try not to be a superstitious man, I will accept a sticky coincidence as a wink from God to say he's got it under control. We chose the name Elizabeth based on a mutual love of a Jane Austen character, long before we knew Elizabeth's condition. But St. Elizabeth, the mother of John the Baptist, is the Catholic patron of difficult pregnancies. We learned of Elizabeth's condition on October 30, the anniversary of my oldest sister's birth, a day before she went to heaven. And Elizabeth was born on the feast of St. Valentine, the patron of those with epilepsy.

God prepares us for our tasks in life, often in ordinary, but sometimes in extraordinary ways. I do not imagine my story will be typical—I don't think there is a typical story in God's plan. God, my creator, spoke to me in the way I would hear, for he knew me. He can speak to each of us differently. But look for the preparation in your life. And trust in him. He will prepare you, if you let him.

Lesson Eight

Begin With Human Dignity
Rejecting "Quality of Life" Ethics

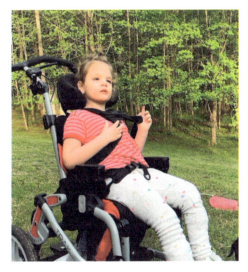

In Elizabeth's room, near her bed, a sign on the wall reads, "Beautiful girl, you can do amazing things." Elizabeth cannot walk or talk. She can barely see. She has low cognitive skills and suffers from epilepsy. But she still dances. She expresses what she wants and needs. She connects to others, and enters into relationship with them.

People often think—and sometime say—a child like this has a "low quality of life." This reflects secular ethics that prioritize *self-autonomy* and *avoidance of pain*. If a person cannot decide for herself, or act on her decisions, or if she experiences regular discomfort or anguish, then her life is not worth living, it is said. But that superficial judgment disregards the child's character. It overlooks her capacity for relationship. In short, it neglects her human dignity.

Self-autonomy is certainly valuable, for it empowers us to pursue what is good, true, and beautiful. But our society treats autonomy as worthy in its own right, reducing the ethics of autonomy to shallow precepts of *tolerance* and *not harming others*, *free choice* and *informed consent*. It is otherwise unconcerned with what we choose.

Pain avoidance provides no better foundation for social ethics. Pain is so woven into the tapestry of our lives that we can only trim it at the edges. Pain is the simplest language of the mind and the body to give lessons to our consciousness. It tells us of injury and weakness, or the absence of something we value. To eliminate pain invites greater harm. Any simple norm differentiating between *good* or *bad* pain, or otherwise explaining what pain should be eliminated, will be either a matter of opinion, or wrong as often as it is right.

Instead, our ethics should be rooted in human dignity. Many, however, don't grasp what *human dignity* means, so secular ethics can highjack the term. "Human" means what it says. We are *homo sapiens*. We embody a particular, living, DNA pattern that passes generation to generation, with marginal variations person to person, shaping our bodies and our capacities. The term "dignity," though, is a little harder to pin down.

Dignity implies an elevated status. But dignity is not vanity, priggishness, or pretension. When someone behaves with dignity, she is not acting as though her surroundings are beneath her. Instead, she arranges her setting, her bearing, her dress, and her manners—in short, everything within her control—to be the best version of what they can be under the circumstance, without being ostentatious or out of place. She may, in fact, disregard arbitrary social norms when they don't serve their purpose. George Washington, it is said, once came to supper in his fine home to find a guest, a lowly veteran of the Revolution. Unaccustomed to formal manners, the visitor lifted the soup bowl to his lips, as he would in his own home. The former President, the general of a nation, the most renowned American of the age, responded by sipping from his own bowl, so the man would not be embarrassed. Washington could conform his bearing to the needs of the moment, prioritizing relationship. This is dignity. In short, the dignified person models what is perfectly appropriate to the precise circumstance of the moment.

Being human, and being alive, is our fundamental circumstance. In our bodies, broken as they may be, we manifest the fundamental truth that we are each appropriately a human being. In this way, by being alive we manifest human dignity. To be a living body—*a living subject*—is to be what a human should be. And being alive is an exceptional state. How little matter in this universe is a part of a self-conscious, living being!

Too often, though, we measure others' value against the rule of normalcy. If a child has a life expectancy of *minutes, hours, days,* or *years,* we compare it to the ordinary life of *seventy, eighty,* or *ninety years.* If a child is *blind,* we focus on the value of *having vision.* If a child *will suffer pain,* we judge that against the ideal of *no pain*. But why should we prefer *no life* to a life of forty-five minutes, if it can't be a life of forty-five million minutes? Do we measure our greatest joys and deepest experiences by minutes? Why should we dread a child's lack of one sensory power, when she is blessed with four more? After all, most matter in this universe has no sensation. Why are we so prejudiced against the thought of another's pain that we would deny the person any opportunity to experience pleasure?

Being a *living human* also means we are in relationship with others, and embracing relationships enhances our human dignity. Relationships are part of the human circumstance—a byproduct of our DNA structure. Our DNA would not have been knit together without our parents' relationship. From the very first moment of our existence, we exist *in relation to another*. We depend on our mothers and other caregivers. We learn through relationships. We supply our wants and our needs through relationships. And when we are disabled, whether through illness, or accident, or congenital anomaly, we depend on relationships.

Through relationships, we exceed our individual limitations. We gain the perspective of others. We benefit from their skills, and reap the fruits of their insights. We fall in love and raise a family. We share a beer with a friend. Through relationships, we survive.

Though our species has caused great evil, together we have also accomplished great good. We have constructed cathedrals and monuments, written great novels and epic histories, learned the mathematics of stars and numbered the pieces of the atom. We have built systems and networks that allow thousands of millions of our species to experience the extraordinary status of *being alive*. In fact, we should be startled we can even acknowledge the evil we have done.

We can think of the human race as a network. Relationships become the conduits of ideas, emotions, goods and services, and the source of inspirations. We can act on one another, for good or for ill. What we communicate to another through a relationship, intentionally or not, may be processed, reshaped, or amplified, and passed on through this network. Information derived from one person or relationship may circulate within the network even after the originator dies or that relationship breaks.

A child like Elizabeth contributes to this network. She has profoundly shaped me, my wife, and our families. She affects those we know, and those we see in passing. She attracts attention, and in her person, *in her body*, she models the dignity of being alive in her circumstance. Through those interactions, her contribution ripples across the network.

And because we live in this human network, affecting one another, human dignity requires us to act appropriately for the occasion. Human dignity is therefore the proper foundation of ethics. Deliberately destroying human life, apart from self-defense or defense of others, would not accord with human dignity. Inflicting torture or slavery diminishes our dignity. Human dignity should shape our treatment of criminals, immigrants, the poor, and the vulnerable. It should motivate our care for the world's environment. It affects sexual ethics, promoting deep intimacy, relationship, and procreation.

And once we prioritize interdependence over self-autonomy, we can find ways to pursue the common good—the social conditions that facilitate human fulfilment, both as individuals and as groups. We can be freed from our narrow interests so as to act selflessly for others.

With human dignity in mind, we can also reengage the problem of pain. Our human condition makes pain unavoidable. Pain will have a role in our life. Reducing and avoiding pain is often fine, but we must integrate the experience of pain into our life in a wholesome manner. This takes character. It takes patience, determination, understanding, self-confidence, and good humor. A capacity for enduring pain empowers us to pursue the good, the true, and the beautiful without reserve.

This choice between secular ethics and human dignity matters. In the Small Room, we knew Elizabeth's diagnosis, but not with certainty her prognosis. The doctor prioritized *pain avoidance* and *autonomy* over *character* and *relationships*. She focused on the worst-case scenario, the outcome most dreadful, as though it were guaranteed. She recommended terminating Elizabeth's life, because autonomy meant my wife could sever this relationship to avoid emotional pain. We need not be burdened with an imperfect child. My religious objection to abortion didn't matter. Our relationships in a faith community didn't matter. And when I resisted further, the physician severed me from the conversation. The physician turned her exclusive attention to Joyce. Autonomy dictated I could not speak for my wife. *Our relationship*, and *my relationship with Elizabeth*, didn't matter. With force of character, Joyce said *no* to ending our daughter's life.

But the conversation with our perinatologist emphasized relationships and character. He spoke of the uncertainty inherent in congenital brain malformations. He told us we had room to hope. He opened to us his own experience as the father of a special needs daughter, speaking of the challenges, the blessings, the sadness, and struggles. In this, we could see his character, and it modelled for us the growth we would need as parents of this little girl. He did not impose a choice, but he allowed us to be in relationship with each other, rather than imposing an artificial autonomy. The diagnosis had not changed, but the acknowledgement that our child had a life to live, and we would learn to be the people to share that life, made all the difference.

So far, this notion of human dignity has not relied on Scripture or religious faith, and purposely so. We need to defend human dignity in a secular world. But for the Christian, the natural truth of human dignity leads us to the bridge of Revelation.

Perhaps no one explains the Christian view of human dignity better than Pope John Paul II in his letter *Evangelium Vitae*, "The Gospel of Life." According to the late Holy Father, the Bible depicts humans as distinct among the creatures of the earth, the pinnacle of God's creative act. *"Let us make human beings in our image, after our likeness."* (Gen. 1:26). *"The LORD God formed man out of dust of the ground and blew into his nostrils the breath of life, and the man became a living being."* (Gen. 2:7). Each person brings a trace of God's glory into the world. Life is a gift. God shares with the person something of God's own life.

Too often we instead think of human beings solely in material terms: a quirk of evolution, the byproduct of his environment. But Scripture shows mankind has primacy over matter. (See Gen. 1:28, 2:5, 15). When Adam encountered the purely material world, he could find no fit helpmate. (Gen. 2:18-20). Only in encountering Eve, in whom the spirit of God also lived, could he exclaim, *"This one, at last, is bone of my bones and flesh of my flesh."* (Gen. 2:23). The material body of Eve revealed a person who was not merely material, a person with whom he could relate. The body is a sign of the person, a *place for the person to be in the world* in order to relate to others, to God, and to the world.

In this encounter between Adam and Eve, we see similarity and difference. Each is human, but they are different, signified in their sexual difference.

God commands the two first parents to fill the earth and subdue it, giving humans a special responsibility to care for life with reverence and love. (Gen. 1:28). Eve's joyful cry on the birth of her first child recognizes this responsibility, for she is only a co-creator. She exclaims, *"I have produced a male child with the help of the LORD."* (Gen. 4:1). God made Adam in God's image, and Adam passed that image to his son. (Gen. 5:1-3).

In short, to be human is to be in this world as a gift from God. To be human is to be a sign of God's glory in the world. To be human is to be human in a particular way, as signified by human sexuality. To be human is to be in relation with others, as signified in the encounter of man and woman. To be human is to be responsible for life.

But sin enters the world. And the first murder follows quickly after the first fall. God's cry to Cain, *"What have you done?"* (Gen. 4:10), echoes through time, addressing each and every attack on life. Too often these attacks arise because we prioritize autonomy and the capacity for communication, thereby demeaning the disabled. We, like Cain, say *"Am I my brother's keeper?"* (Gen. 4:8). The late Pope responds with a resounding *"Yes!"* "God entrusts us to one another," John Paul says. (*Evangelium Vitae*, 19). We abuse the freedom of choice when we, like Cain, divorce ourselves from relationship. We abuse freedom when we divorce ourselves from objective truth.

But self-autonomy has become our goal, because we lost the sense of God's presence in each and every person. We see the human person as only *a thing in this world*, without a transcendent character. His life is his property, his to control and to manipulate. *Having* becomes more important than *being*. We reject suffering as useless.

Yet even in our fallen state, God does not abandon us, and our dignity, though marred, has not been eradicated. Through the Exodus, God shows that the dignity of the person should shape the social order, and he offers an enslaved people the chance to devise a cultural identity informed by this truth. Israel tries and fails, tries and fails. Yet the Wisdom literature shows Israel's capacity to reverence human dignity, rooted in man's relationship with God. *"You formed my inmost being; you knit me in my mother's womb. I praise you, because I am wonderfully made."* (Ps. 139:13-14). *"What is man that you are mindful of him, and a son of man that you care for him? Yet you have made him little less than a god, crowned him with glory and honor. You have given him rule over the works of your hands, put all things at his feet."* (Ps. 8:5-7). *"God did not make death, nor does he rejoice in the destruction of the living. For he fashioned all things that they may have being."* (Wis. 1:13-14). *"For God formed us to be imperishable; the image of his own nature he made us."* (Wis. 2:23).

But the meaning of human dignity remained partially veiled in the Old Testament. And then Christ came. *God* came into his creation *as a human being*. His divinity elevated the human form. We are the kind of being God became to sanctify creation. And in and through Christ, God reveals his internal life as a trinity of Divine Persons. God's life *is relationship*. Now we can understand better how the duality of the sexes, with the natural capacity to join together in a life-producing one-flesh union, images the life of God. Now we can understand better the priority of relationships over individuality.

Christ came as a child—a vulnerable, dependent child. He depended on the aid of others. His life fell under mortal threat nearly from the beginning, as Herod sought to destroy him, forcing his family to flee to Egypt. (Matt. 2:13-23). And so, he knew what it was to be vulnerable.

In his ministry, Christ showed the dignity of every person through his special care for the poor and the marginalized, the sick and the disabled. He says, *"I came so that they may have life and have it more abundantly."* (John 10:10). He tells his followers, *"I am the way and the truth and the life."* (John 14:6). He says, *"I am the resurrection and the life; whoever believes in me, even if he dies, will live, and everyone who lives and believes in me will never die."* (John 11:25-26). This life is not simply life in time, life as we know it in this world, but an outpouring of God's eternal life through relationship with him. Christ says, *"For this is the will of my Father, that everyone who sees the Son and believes in him may have eternal life, and I shall raise him on the last day."* (John 6:40). Peter acknowledges this, too: *"Master, to whom shall we go? You have the words of eternal life. We have come to believe and are convinced that you are the Holy One of God."* (John 6:68-69).

Pope John Paul II captures the majesty of Christ's teaching in these words:

> *Man is called to a fullness of life which far exceeds the dimensions of his earthly existence, because it consists in sharing the very life of God. The loftiness of this supernatural vocation reveals the greatness and the inestimable value of human life even in its temporal phase. Life in time, in fact, is the fundamental condition, the initial stage and an integral part of the entire unified process of human existence. It is a process which, unexpectedly and undeservedly, is enlightened by the promise and renewed by the gift of divine life, which will reach its full realization in eternity (cf. 1 Jn 3:1-2). At the same time, it is precisely this supernatural calling which highlights the relative character of each individual's earthly life. After all, life on earth is not an "ultimate" but a "penultimate" reality; even so, it remains a sacred reality entrusted to us, to be preserved with a sense of responsibility and brought to perfection in love and in the gift of ourselves to God and to our brothers and sisters. (Evangelium Vitae, 2).*

In short, human dignity arises not simply because God is the source of human life, but also because God unites himself to us in time and eternity.

And then, at the culmination of his ministry, Christ surrenders his life. He embraces some of the worst suffering possible, so that everyone who suffers might know that God is with them. Christ's willingness to surrender his precious life for the salvation of man proves more than anything the dignity of human life. *"[Y]ou were ransomed from your futile conduct, handed on by your ancestors, not with perishable things such as silver or gold, but with the precious blood of Christ, as of a spotless unblemished lamb."* (1 Pt. 1:18-19).

But death is not the end of the story. Christ rises from the dead. Because he rose, we can trust his earlier promise: *"I am the resurrection and the life; he who believes in me, though he die, yet shall he live, and whoever lives and believes in me shall never die."* (John 11:25-26). This promise of eternal resurrection explains the works of healing both Christ and his apostles performed. These healings were a sign of Christ's forgiveness of sin. By turning to God for forgiveness of sins, and opening our hearts to his mercy, we prepare ourselves to receive the gift of resurrection and eternal life. Death then becomes the pathway into life.

I hope in the resurrection. My faith teaches that the resurrection is not simply a feel-good promise, or an expressive way to speak of a spiritual encounter with God. It is a bodily resurrection. Somehow, someway, our bodies will be reconstituted into a form that is at once glorified but still distinctly individual, still sharing in the continuity of our present identity. I cannot prove or even justify this through secular reasoning. But I hope in the resurrection, resting on the promise of Christ. And when that day comes, I will seek out my daughter Elizabeth, my daughter who had a broken brain in this life, and I will embrace her in her glory.

I think she will bear in heaven the marks of her suffering in life, like the image in Revelation of the Lamb who was slain. (Rev. 5:6). Those marks will be elevated in beauty, for through them she manifests God's glory in the world, by being a sign of contradiction. In a world obsessed with utility, her life does not make sense. In a world preoccupied by autonomy, her

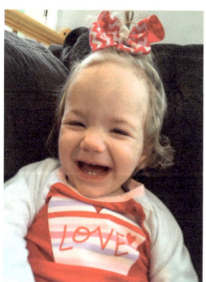

dependence seems a burden. In a world that despises suffering, her pains are absurd. And yet she lives. And she dances. And she communicates. And she loves. She embodies the image of God. She brings a trace of God's glory into this world.

Yet I hope somehow I will encounter Elizabeth beyond her limitations, beyond her disabilities. I want my sightless child to see my face in heaven. I want my voiceless child to speak to me. I want her to understand what I say. I want to tell her it has been a privilege to be her father.

Beautiful girl, you can do amazing things. In your body, in your way of being human, you encounter this world as no one else can. You have unique experiences, and unique relationships. And through those relationships you teach love and patience, and joy in the simple things. You teach us our limits are far beyond our expectations. And we carry these lessons into the world. Your impact cannot be measured by your degree of autonomy, and it is not negated by your suffering. *You make God's glory present in this world.* Even with your broken body and brain, you are a place where we encounter God.

Beautiful girl, you can do amazing things.

Lesson Nine

I May Be Broken
Encountering Our Limits

In the Shenandoah Valley, in western Virginia, lies a small Catholic college, called Christendom. When I attended Christendom, the college had fewer than four hundred students. I did not know everyone, but I recognized everyone's face. And everyone recognized Coach Vander Woude.

As the athletics director and the men's basketball coach, Tom Vander Woude was the heart of Christendom's sports program. He was fierce with his team, but he never attracted attention. His players loved him.

And if you saw Coach, you'd also see his youngest son nearby, walking behind or shooting hoops in the gym. His son had Down's syndrome. And when I think of a man who has modeled fatherhood to a special needs child, I think of Coach Vander Woude. Not only for the way he lived and made his son a part of our community, but for the way he died.

The Vander Woudes lived on a farm. Some years after I graduated, Coach's son fell through the boards covering an old septic tank on the property. Unable to pull him out from above, and seeing his son struggling in the deep mire, Coach Vander Woude jumped into the pit. In the muck and the filth, he lifted his son high, until the rescue team pulled the boy out. But they could not save Coach Vander Woude.

Occasionally I hear that we are not going to die for our Christian beliefs, at least in this country. I think of Coach Vander Woude. Coach Vander Woude believed in the dignity of life. He believed in the dignity of his son. He lived what he believed, and he died for his beliefs.

As parents of special needs children, we surrender control, and we find joy in our suffering. We love fiercely. We connect with others, and we accept the preparation we receive. But a shadow always looms at the edge of our consciousness, a sense of vulnerability. We know someday we may face a challenge beyond our endurance. This is not anxiety or depression, but sober realism. *Someday, we may be broken.*

My family is fragile. My child may suffer an injury or medical setback any day. And if someone else in my family suffers a severe accident or illness, the burden may be overwhelming. We have already experienced challenges that pushed us to the edge. We know we can be broken.

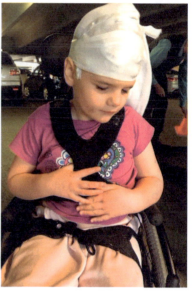

I write these words from the emergency room at the hospital. Elizabeth has been vomiting all week, without a clear reason. Meanwhile, Joyce is thirty-nine weeks pregnant and may go into labor at any time. It's going to be a long night. It's going to be a long week.

People often say God will not give us more than we can handle. I don't believe it. I look at Christ on the cross, crying out to his Father, *"My God, my God! Why have you forsaken me?"* (Matt. 27:46, Mark 15:34). Are these not the words of a broken man? And yet he can also say in the end, *"Father, into your hands I commend my spirit."* (Luke 23:46). It is, in a way, a broken *hallelujah*.

Hallelujah is a beautiful prayer. Derived from Hebrew, the word means *Sing praise to Yahweh!* The "-jah" is a shortened form of God's name, *I AM*, as communicated to Moses. (Ex. 3:14). We often forget that "God" is not God's name, and through a tradition of reverencing the precious name of God with silence, we grow distant from him. But the *hallelujah* invites us back into relationship with a God who has a name.

Hallelujah is a song, begging to be sung. It is the Spirit swelling within the soul and escaping as a long, melodious sound. And Revelation tells us this song echoes in the court of heaven. (Rev. 19:1-6). Seventeen Psalms open with *Hallelujah!*, and the last words of the last psalm summarizes the lesson, *"Let everything that has breath give praise to the LORD! Hallelujah!"* (Ps. 150:6).

Hallelujah comes easy in a moment of ecstatic joy. At Easter or Christmas, *Hallelujah!* seems appropriate. But if everything that breathes should praise Yahweh, the *hallelujah* should escape our lips in good times and bad, in sickness and in health. We should praise *I AM* in moments of distress. We should praise *I Am* in our moments of brokenness. A broken *hallelujah* may be what matters the most in the end.

And we can be broken. Scripture does not promise that God will give us only what we can bear. Scripture only promises we won't be *tempted* beyond what we can bear. (1 Cor. 10:13). We will not be forced into sin, but our bodies may be broken, and God may allow it. Our minds may be broken, and God may allow it. Our relationships may be broken, and God may allow it.

As proof, we need only to look at the story of Job. Job was an innocent man, not deserving reproach. (Job 1:1). But Satan thought Job was good only because things were easy for him. Satan tells God, *"Have you not surrounded him and his family and all that he has with your protection? You have blessed the work of his hands, and his livestock are spread over the land. But now put forth your hand and touch all that he has, and surely he will curse you to your face."* And God allows his faithful servant to be tested. (Job 1:6-12).

In a moment, Job loses his wealth and his children. Yet he falls to the ground and worships God. *"Naked I came forth from my mother's womb,"* he prays, *"and naked shall I go back there. The LORD gave and the LORD has taken away; blessed be the name of the LORD!"* (Job 1:21). He sings *hallelujah* in his distress. He is not broken.

But Satan returns to God, offering a new challenge. *"All that a man has he will give for his life. But put forth your hand and touch his bone and his flesh. Then surely he will curse you to your face."* And God allows his faithful servant to be tested.

Boils appear on Job's flesh *"from the soles of his feet to the crown of his head."* (Job 2:1-6). This new struggle provokes discord between Job and his wife. His wife, too, has lost all the children she bore, and in her frustration and grief, she cries, *"Curse God and die!"* Job responds, *"You speak as foolish women do. We accept good things from God; should we not accept evil?"* (Job 2:9-10).

Yet Job continues to suffer. His friends come to him, and Job suffers on. (Job 2:11-13). But the pain and frustration become too much, and Job curses the day of his birth, repudiating the value of his life. (Job 3). In a long speech, Job's friend suggests that Job should simply pray and God will take the troubles away. (Job 4-5).

This recommendation to "just pray" offends Job, and he responds sharply, cataloguing his sufferings. (Job 6-7). Another friend speaks, encouraging Job not to give in to despair. (Job 8). He says if Job is righteous, he should pray, and God will take away his sufferings. Job does not believe he sinned, and so he cannot repent. He bitterly demands that God justify these sufferings. (Job 9-10). The third friend reprimands Job, assured that

God must see some hidden sin. (Job 11). Job grows hostile toward his friends, accusing them of thinking themselves better and wiser than him. (Job 12-13). He insists God does as he wishes in the affairs of man. (Job 13:21-24). He wishes to be forgotten by God, until God's wrath against him abates. (Job 14:13).

Through five more speeches, Job's friends try to persuade him to repent. They recount in colorful terms what evildoers suffer if they do not change their ways. Job criticizes his friends, lamenting his sufferings, and demanding answers of God. Finally he swears oaths of his innocence, and his friends fall silent. (Job 15-31).

This story depicts a man broken by his suffering. In place of his humble song of submission at the beginning of the story, Job has become a bitter man. But he has not rejected God. He instead confronts God. He criticizes God's choices. He demands answers. But he has not rejected God.

God finally replies directly to Job. (Job 38-39). God offers no answers, but presents questions that show his overarching power and wisdom:

> *Where were you when I founded the earth?*
> *Tell me, if you have understanding.*
> *Who determined its size? Surely you know?*
> *Who stretched out the measuring line for it?*
>
> *Into what were its pedestals sunk,*
> *and who laid its cornerstone,*
> *While the morning stars sang together*
> *and all the sons of God shouted for joy?* (Job 38:4-7).

On and on, God continues, humbling Job. When at last God pauses for an answer, Job demurs. *"Look, I am of little account,"* the suffering man says, *"what can I answer you? I put my hand over my mouth."* (Job 40:4). But God is not satisfied with silence. (Job 40-41). He presses on, until Job speaks again, finally responding as he should.

> *I know that you can do all things,*
> *and that no purpose of yours can be hindered.*
> . . . .
> *I have spoken but did not understand;*
> *things too marvelous for me, which I did not know.*
> . . . .
> *By hearsay I had heard of you,*
> *but now my eye has seen you.*
> *Therefore I disown what I have said,*
> *and repent in dust and ashes.* (Job 42:2-6).

This is Job's broken *hallelujah*—an acknowledgement of God's power, an admission of Job's own failings, and remorse. In his sufferings he had challenged God. But God recognizes Job was driven by prolonged, agonizing pain, and God does not hold it against him. Job is a broken man, but he has not rejected God. Instead, God turns to Job's accusers, his three friends, and proclaims his anger toward them. *"You have not spoken rightly concerning me, as has my servant Job."* He tells them to sacrifice and to petition Job to pray on their behalf, for God will show favor to Job. (Job 42:7-8). And he restores to Job prosperity and family, and gives him a long life. (Job 42:10-17).

We can be broken. Like Job, we can be brought to the point of challenging God, or cursing our sufferings and repudiating the gift of life. But we learn from Job that God paints the story of our life on a canvas much broader than our vision, and our brokenness may mar our experience without disrupting the portrait. Being broken, being truly broken, is not a sin.

Job shows us that a broken body can break a spirit and fracture relationships. Our body, spirit, and relationships are woven together, and breaking one of these threads will strain the other two.

Parenting Elizabeth makes my body more prone to be broken. She often injures us through bites, scratches, slaps, or kicks. Lifting, carrying, and manipulating her body takes a toll on me. It may break me someday.

Parenting Elizabeth challenges my spirit. Stress overwhelms me at times. I try not to imagine the future, deliberately blocking it from my mind, because I am not yet the man who can handle a fully grown woman with these conditions. It is something that might break me.

But my greatest fear—the shadow at the edge of my consciousness—is the fear of broken relationships. My time with Elizabeth will end with her dying while I live, or me dying while she lives. What will happen to Elizabeth when my wife and I are gone? Will someone be there to care for her? To play music and sing? To sit with her? To suffer for her? I fear facing my death not knowing what will come of Elizabeth. It might break me.

On the other hand, I also fear what Elizabeth's death may do for me and for my family. How would we handle Elizabeth's death? Most marriages survive the death of a child—only about one in six marriages fail. But I cannot know my marriage will survive. And if it does, how will our relationship change? How will we each handle the grief? What will Elizabeth's death mean for our children? I cannot know. And it may break me.

I am blessed that I do not live with more fears. Many families know greater stress than mine, like *How will we afford the treatment or the equipment we need? How will we afford childcare? Can we keep our jobs? What if we become pregnant again? What if we have another child? What if that child has special needs? Will I live all my life as a caregiver?* Any one of these concerns could break someone, and one concern usually invites others.

As I write this, though, I am looking at my daughter, in the emergency room. All the tests say she is healthy, but she is still vomiting brown bile, and has been all day.

A pediatric specialist stops by. I tell him what brought us in, for the umpteenth time. As I explain Elizabeth's history, I see my daughter rigid and shaking. She is seizing, like I have only seen once or twice before. She continues to seize. Her heart rate climbs to three beats a second. On and on she seizes. Doctors and nurses crowd the room. Oxygen lines appear. The ER specialist quietly takes command. A nurse runs dosing calculations and reports to the doctor, before pushing a drug by IV. The seizure continues for another minute, then two.

The thought surfaces in my mind—*This could be how it ends. A seizure in the emergency room, and the doctors can't save her.* I suppress the thought, fighting to stay present in the moment.

A half hour later, Elizabeth sleeps. Oxygen still hisses through the tubes. My body shakes, but I know the adrenaline will burn off soon. Still, I suppress the creeping shadow, for now. I will wait until later to feel my vulnerability.

We can't escape the fact that we can break. We shouldn't pretend it's impossible. Admitting we can all break is an act of mercy. After all, if we say God will never give us more than we can bear, we demean those who have broken under their load. Like Job's friends, we blame the broken man.

Instead, we must accept our vulnerability. Surrendering control, connecting with others, and living in mercy helps us to push back the breaking point, but we parents of special needs children should also consider how we can sing *hallelujah* even if we find ourselves broken.

Picture in your mind a beautiful image: the Niagara Falls or the Grand Canyon, the mighty oceans teaming with life, or the wonderful animals of the forests and plains. Our capacity to perceive beauty reflects the remarkable quality of human subjectivity. We are material beings in a material world, but we are beings with subjectivity. A world without humanity is qualitatively different than a world with humanity, for our subjectivity permits us to proclaim the truth, celebrate the beautiful, and serve the good. This is a human capacity, a way we manifest human dignity.

Through our subjectivity, we can marvel at being. We exist. And it is not simply *our* existence that is marvelous, but *being* itself. Being is wonderful. It is the wonder of the great *I AM*, the source and foundation of existence. The act we call *being*, taken in itself, is God. He is *I AM*.

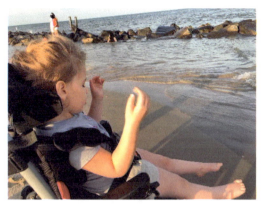

God is the foundation of being, and because of this, God is praiseworthy. Praising God is the appropriate human response to the recognition that we are alive—we participate in the being of *I AM*. This call to praise God exists irrespective of our condition or circumstance. The qualitative difference between *being alive* and *not being* renders the differences in our conditions or circumstances during life insignificant by comparison.

We have been given time for praising God, and *this time—while we are alive*—this is it. We praise God not only through our words, but also through our deeds. Parenting a child praises God, for it brings another person into being and raises her to praise *I AM*. Parenting a child with special needs praises *I AM* in a special way, for these children manifest the value of simply being, of simply participating in the life of *I AM*.

When we find ourselves broken through our care of a person with special needs, our *pain and suffering* is an *hallelujah*. The choices that have brought us to that point have etched our praise into our body, into our emotions, and into our relationships. We are material beings. We have limits. We don't control everything. We can be broken, and still we chose to praise God through our care of our special needs children, at great cost to ourselves. Our suffering, like the sufferings of Christ, become the *hallelujah*.

Living and singing *hallelujah* now, through the care of our children with special needs—*now, while sacrifice is a joy*—builds within us the capacity to sing a broken *hallelujah*. Job's praise and sacrifice to *I AM* before and during his sufferings prepared him for his prolonged agony. Likewise, Coach Vander Woude made an *hallelujah* of his life, giving it up to save his son, but Coach Vander Woude could do it only because he had already sacrificed himself for his son *ten thousand times before*.

Christ points the way forward for the broken soul through his plea on the Cross—*"My God, My God! Why have you forsaken me?"* (Matt. 27:46, Mark 15:34). This is a reference to Psalm 22, a great psalm of suffering, a psalm in four parts:

Part I

My God, my God, why have you abandoned me?
Why so far from my call for help,
from my cries of anguish?
My God, I call by day, but you do not answer;
by night, but I have no relief.

Yet you are enthroned as the Holy One;
you are the glory of Israel.
In you our fathers trusted;
they trusted and you rescued them.

To you they cried out and they escaped;
in you they trusted and were not disappointed.
But I am a worm, not a man,
scorned by men, despised by the people.

All who see me mock me;
they curl their lips and jeer;
they shake their heads at me:
"He relied on the LORD—let him deliver him;
if he loves him, let him rescue him."

For you drew me forth from the womb,
made me safe at my mother's breasts.
Upon you I was thrust from the womb;
since my mother bore me you are my God.

Do not stay far from me,
for trouble is near,
and there is no one to help.

This is the image of a broken man. We feel a profound separation from God in a time of great anguish, whether from a broken body, a broken spirit, or a broken relationship. Despite prayer, the suffering goes on.

We can sense a flickering of faith and looming temptation to doubt. Stories of God's goodness carry us only so far in the face of suffering. Hope struggles against anger. *If God exists, is God powerless, malicious, or indifferent?*

Past faithfulness becomes a source of humiliation. We believed, and we still want to believe. But where is our champion in this moment of need?

We see in these Old Testament lines the same distress we experience in our life. But unlike the psalmist, we can take comfort in Christ, who came in response to this prayer. God, in fact, did not stay far from me, but came into creation to rescue me.

Part II

Many bulls surround me;
fierce bulls of Bashan encircle me.
They open their mouths against me,
lions that rend and roar.

Like water my life drains away;
all my bones are disjointed.
My heart has become like wax,
it melts away within me.

As dry as a potsherd is my throat;
my tongue cleaves to my palate;
you lay me in the dust of death.

Dogs surround me;
a pack of evildoers closes in on me.
They have pierced my hands and my feet
I can count all my bones.

They stare at me and gloat;
they divide my garments among them;
for my clothing they cast lots.

But you, LORD, do not stay far off;
my strength, come quickly to help me.

Deliver my soul from the sword,
my life from the grip of the dog.
Save me from the lion's mouth,
my poor life from the horns of wild bulls.

Fear for the future consumes our attention, in the face of physical and spiritual threats. All that we love in life slips away. Death, or despair, seems imminent.

We have faced struggles before, but this is far, far beyond our strength. We cannot go on like this!

There is no comfort in anything or anyone. We feel isolation.

God, please help! I believe in you!

This imagery connects us to the suffering psalmist, and through the psalmist to all humanity. Yet it also connects us to Christ, suffering on the cross, crying out with a parched tongue, *"I thirst!"* (Cf. John 19:28).

Part III

Then I will proclaim your name to my brethren;
in the assembly I will praise you:

"You who fear the LORD, give praise!
All descendants of Jacob, give honor;
show reverence, all descendants of Israel!

For he has not spurned or disdained
the misery of this poor wretch,
Did not turn away from me,
but heard me when I cried out.

I will offer praise in the great assembly;
my vows I will fulfill before those who fear him.
The poor will eat their fill;
those who seek the LORD will offer praise.
May your hearts enjoy life forever!"

We wish to bargain with God, though we know that is not how it works. So instead, we make promises that presuppose he will save us.

We try to build our faith by remembering what we were told about God's mercy to the faithful in times gone by. We try to summon within us belief in a loving God, struggling to give sincere praise to *I AM*. We try to imagine how we will celebrate God's mercy when he saves us from our distress.

"May your hearts enjoy life forever"—An idealistic hope for a man in a moment of distress, yet a hope fulfilled in Christ's redemptive gift of his eternal life.

Part IV

All the ends of the earth
will remember and turn to the LORD;
All the families of nations
will bow low before him.
For kingship belongs to the LORD,
the ruler over the nations.

All who sleep in the earth
will bow low before God;

All who have gone down into the dust
will kneel in homage.
And I will live for the LORD;
my descendants will serve you.

The generation to come will be told of the LORD,
that they may proclaim to a people yet unborn
the deliverance you have brought.

The flame of hope flickers, but does not go out. We reconcile ourselves to our condition, broken as we may be. We wrest our attention from the threats we face and suffering we experience to the universal and eternal dominion of *I AM*. Just as Job was able to accept his suffering in light of God's all-encompassing providence, so too we can accept suffering and brokenness, praising God, in Christ, with an *Hallelujah!*

Raising a child with special needs is a great challenge. You may be broken. I may be broken. But we will live for *I AM*. We can be reconciled with brokenness and allow our sufferings—like those of Coach Vander Woude—to praise him. Our brokenness will be our *hallelujah*.

Three days have passed since Elizabeth's severe seizure. She lies in the hospital bed after a mostly restless night, listening to some music. She has had no more seizures, and the vomiting is under control for now. We should be going home today. Elizabeth's brother has not come yet, but he probably will soon. Someday, I may be broken by this challenge of parenting Elizabeth. But not today. *Hallelujah!*

Lesson Ten

Walk with Those Who Walk with God
Living in the Mystical Body

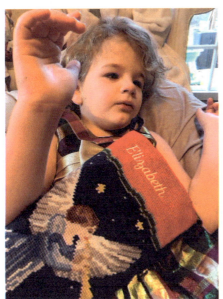

I sit with Elizabeth on the floor, with her evening pills at hand—six of them—and a banana to coax them down. Bedtime approaches. My daughter lays calmly across my lap, enjoying home life after days in the hospital. Joyce joins us, touching Elizabeth's hand. Elizabeth grabs her mother's fingers, delighting in the connection. It is time for our evening prayers.

I call my five-year-old and the two-year-old. They are playing, and do not respond immediately. I call again. I know our prayers will be interrupted with bathroom breaks, letting the dog out, distractions, and scolding, but still we will teach our children to pray. We will teach them to walk with God.

Elizabeth cannot pray with us, but she is with us when we pray. Scripture shows the merit of praying with and for one another. Job's friends must ask Job to pray for them. (Job 42:8). And Paul tells Timothy, *"I ask that supplications, prayers, petitions, and thanksgivings be offered for everyone, for kings and for all in authority, that we may lead a quiet and tranquil life in all devotion and dignity. This is good and pleasing to God our savior."* (1 Tim. 2:1-3).

Christ himself shows the value of praying for another, in a story recorded by both Mark and Luke. (Mark 2:1-12; Luke 5:17-26). Jesus and his disciples were in Capernaum. People filled the house, including Pharisees and scribes from distant cities. No one else could fit, even around the door. And so, four men climbed to the roof of the house. They broke through the ceiling, and lowered their paralyzed friend using ropes, laying his stretcher at the feet of Jesus.

And Jesus looked up. He looked *up*, at this man's friends—both Matthew and Luke record this. And when Jesus saw his companions' faith, he said to the paralytic, *"Your sins are forgiven."* Then, Jesus shows the scribes and the Pharisees that he was not blaspheming, that he could forgive sins, by telling the incapacitated man to rise and go home. The man did so, astonishing the crowd, who glorified God.

Christ showed mercy to this man because of his companions, men who proved their love and faith by carrying him through the streets, climbing a wall, and tearing through a ceiling, to place the man in Christ's presence. Think of the passion that moved these men! Their outrageous determination! And so we, like these companions of the paralytic, pray with and for our daughter, placing our child before Christ, confident in the Lord's mercy.

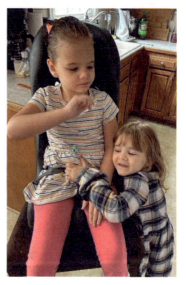

God entrusts us to one another in this life. As we walk with Our Lord, he expects us to be with one another. He expects us to carry each other if we must, climbing walls and tearing through ceilings. For some reason, he has entrusted the body and soul of this child not only to me and my wife, but also to her siblings, and to our families, our friends, our parish, and the broader community. Together, we are to walk with her, walking with him.

Tonight, as always, we pray for those who walk with us. We pray for each member of our family by name, and we ask specifically for what they need. We pray for our aunts, our uncles, our cousins, and our grandmas and grandpas. We ask God to bless the doctors, nurses, therapists, teachers, and nannies who have helped our children. We pray for the leaders of our Church and our parish. I pray for my wife and our marriage, and that we and our children will see heaven someday. We invite our daughters to add their intentions. Our five-year-old—a child of habit—offers the same prayer we have heard every day this summer, for her kindergarten class. Our two-year-old adds her list: "Emmah and Ickie." "Ickie" means our nanny, Ms. Vickie. "Emmah" is her name for a furry red monster from television.

St. Paul captures this spirit of living for one another through the imagery of the Mystical Body of Christ. In his letter to the Romans (12:1, 4-8), he writes:

> *I urge you therefore, brothers, by the mercies of God, to offer your bodies as a living sacrifice, holy and pleasing to God, your spiritual worship.*
>
> *. . . . For as in one body we have many parts, and all the parts do not have the same function, so we, though many, are one body in Christ and individually parts of one another.*
>
> *Since we have gifts that differ according to the grace given to us, let us exercise them: if prophecy, in proportion to the faith; if ministry, in ministering; if one is a teacher, in teaching; if one exhorts, in exhortation; if one contributes, in generosity; if one is over others, with diligence; if one does acts of mercy, with cheerfulness.*

Put another way, our mission in life is not to be our true self for the sake of self-fulfillment. Instead, we are called to serve others. The prophet does not prophesy for himself. The minister does not minister for himself. So, too, the teacher, the one who exhorts, the contributor, the leader, and those who act with mercy. All we have been given is for service of others, to build the body of Christ. Our whole life, our whole body, our whole being, are to be sacrificed in service of others, as worship to God.

This call to total and complete sacrifice in service of others should both challenge and comfort us. It challenges us because we are not allowed to hold anything back. We cannot carve something out as our own. God does not take too much when he takes it all.

But this universal Christian vocation should also comfort us parents of special needs children. We are part of something bigger. Our special children are part of something bigger. Our children may not prophesy or minister, teach or exhort. But their lives and sufferings, their smiles and tears, are all integrated as offerings in the Mystical Body of Christ. Elizabeth partakes in the mystery of Christ's redemptive work. And therefore my service to her—however great the challenge is—builds up the Body of Christ.

Moreover, the universal call of service comforts us because all who walk with Christ are to be there for us and our special children. I can and must rely on others. I can and must rest in the generosity of others. I can and must receive what others offer as their part in building up the body of Christ.

When someone goes the extra mile out of love of Christ, I should not feel as though we have imposed. I should feel gratitude and know we stand together in the Body of Christ.

But the Mystical Body of Christ joins us to more than just the Christians of our present age. It joins us to the faithful who have gone to their eternal reward. Christ says his Father *"is not God of the dead, but of the living, for to him all are alive."* (Luke 20:38). Abraham, Isaac, and Jacob, and all the saints are alive in God and in the Body of Christ. Walking with Christ gives us the great privilege of walking with those great men and women who also walk with Christ. We can rely on the saints to help carry our load, turning to them for aid, comfort, and inspiration. We know from John's Revelation that the saints offer prayers to the Lord. These prayers are *"golden bowls of incense"* before the Lamb. (Rev. 8:4). Certainly those may include prayers from the saints offered on our behalf.

For this reason, each night our family calls on particular saints by name to "pray for us, guide us, protect us, and keep us." This litany is not meant to be prattled like a magic incantation or a memory game. These are real people—real personalities—who walked with God in joy and in pain, in times of stress and times of serenity. We say their names, and when the chaos of family life does not intrude, I try to connect with the living memory of each.

For my eldest daughter, we pray first to St. Elizabeth, the mother of John the Babtist. Like Sarah, Rebekah, Rachel, Samson's mother, and Hannah before her, she suffered the embarrassment of being childless after many years of marriage. (Luke 1:7). Yet her name means *"God's promise."* An angel appeared to her husband Zechariah and promised a child, but Zechariah doubted and demanded a sign. God fulfilled Zechariah's request by rendering him mute. (Luke 1:10-20). Can we imagine Elizabeth meeting her spouse after this angelic encounter? What could he communicate to her? After all, we do not know if Elizabeth could read. Elizabeth must have worried as she discovered her pregnancy, now that her husband was disabled. But we see joy when her cousin, Mary, came to help her in her need. Elizabeth became the first of our race to vocally acknowledge Mary's child, Jesus, as Lord. (Luke 1:42-43).

When Elizabeth delivered her child, she resisted the pressure of neighbors and relatives and insisted on naming him John. (Luke 1:58-61). We imagine Zechariah directed her to use this name. But perhaps Zechariah could not communicate to her. Perhaps God used the challenges of her life to inspire this strong woman to select this name, a name that expresses what this child means to her: *"Yahweh has shown favor."* And, of course, this child would proclaim the favor God has shown to all mankind, preparing the way for Christ.

We pray to St. Elizabeth to strengthen my daughter and our family in adversity. My child Elizabeth is God's promise to me. God cultivated in my heart years before my daughter was born the expectation that I would face a great challenge, a challenge that could shake me to the core. My daughter Elizabeth fulfilled God's promise, and I am so much the better for it. My Elizabeth suffers a condition that lessens her in the eyes of society, as did St. Elizabeth. She has the strength of St. Elizabeth—determination under pressure, long-suffering, and joy. Through her, I can see God has shown me his favor.

We also pray to St. Thérèse of Lisieux, the Little Flower. Born in France in 1873, she had four older sisters. Though her family spoiled her, it did not spoil her temperament. Her mother died when Thérèse was four, and her sisters—her surrogate mothers—later joined a cloistered convent. Though she suffered through these losses, she learned she could forget her sufferings by dedicating herself to acts of charity. At fifteen, she too joined the Carmelite convent.

Though Thérèse dreamt of becoming a missionary, she realized she could accomplish as much for distant souls by engaging in every small act throughout the day with great charity and love. This became her "Little Way" of sanctity. She died from tuberculosis when she was twenty-four, but not before she wrote her memoirs at the direction of her sister, who had become her religious superior. The book, *The Story of a Soul*, led to her being named a Doctor of the Catholic Church, in recognition of her contribution to Christian spirituality.

Elizabeth, I know, will never do anything great in the eyes of the world. But she has been integrated into the Mystical Body of Christ by baptism, and Christ can use her sufferings for the benefit of others, just as he accepted St. Thérèse's offerings for the benefit of the Church. Like St. Thérèse, my Elizabeth tolerates so much, forgetting her sufferings through music or cuddles with someone she loves. This is my daughter's little way. We pray that the Little Flower will take Elizabeth by the hand and lead her through this life and into a place in heaven.

We pray for the intercession of another Therese as well—St. Teresa of Calcutta, better known as Mother Teresa. Born in 1910 in Albania, she joined the Sisters of Loreto in Ireland at eighteen, offering herself as a missionary. The convent sent her to India, and with her first profession in 1931, she took the name Teresa, with St. Thérèse of Lisieux as her patroness.

Mother Teresa became a teacher in Calcutta, but in 1946, she felt what she later described as a call within the call, a prompting from Christ to serve the poor beyond the walls of her convent. She received permission to leave her order, and in 1950, she founded the Missionaries of Charity. She became a beggar for herself and for those in need whom she encountered. In time, she organized hospice care for the needy and for lepers, and homes for orphans and homeless youth. By her death in 1997, nearly 4,000 sisters and more than 350 brothers were serving the poor as Missionaries of Charity.

For me, no one models fierce love better than Mother Teresa——but not fierceness of anger so much as a profound and unrelenting determination in the face of human suffering. She was not a timid soul. All who crossed her orbit have stories of how she drew forth, through high expectation, example, and force of will, a degree of charity they were not otherwise prepared to offer. On the crucifix in each convent chapel for the Missionaries of Charity hangs a sign: *"I Thirst."* This reminds the sisters of Christ's words, expressing both a physical thirst and a thirst for souls. (John 19:28). And the sisters seek to quench Christ's thirst by caring for the poor, knowing *"Whatever you do for the least of these, you do for me."* (See Matt. 25:40). By giving a drink, or food, or clothes, or shelter, or medical care to those in need, they come as close as they might in this present day to giving Christ a drink in his sufferings. And through their example of charity and their proclamation of the Gospel in word and deed, they also quench Christ's thirst for souls.

I see in Elizabeth the same fierce determination Mother Teresa exhibited in her own sufferings. Who is not struck by the image of Mother Teresa, a frail woman, with a body and hands bent through long years of physical service, praying the rosary or reaching out to help a starving or sick person in need? I cannot imagine the physical and emotional sufferings she went through in her ministry, and I see in Elizabeth the same capacity for joy despite profound and prolonged suffering. I pray to Mother Teresa because I need to be guided by her model of charity in parenting Elizabeth.

I have grown close to these pious women through my years of devotion on Elizabeth's behalf. Their example and stories help to orient my service of Elizabeth, as I ask them to petition God for her.

But we solicit the intercession of one more saint above all others, for she of all people walked with Jesus most during his life. As a young woman, she received her invitation to participate in Jesus's ministry. She was with him before he chose his disciples, and she was with him through his Crucifixion. Then she was with the disciples when they received the Holy Spirit. St. Paul tells us to *"offer your bodies as a living sacrifice, holy and pleasing to God, your spiritual worship."* (Rom. 12:1). This extraordinary woman literally gave Christ her body. She accepted, as an unmarried woman, an unplanned pregnancy of a special child. She was engaged to be wed, but her fiancé was not the father. Under the law, she could be killed by stoning if her fiancé denounced her, yet she continued in carrying the pregnancy, with faith in God's plan, faith greater than even Abraham's.

And God was not gentle with her. To give this child a chance at life, she and her new husband had to walk away from all that they knew on a moment's notice and resettle their lives far from the place they called home. When they finally returned to their home country, they chose a new city to keep their child safe. Their quiet home life was still punctuated with crises, such as when the child eloped during a pilgrimage, missing for days in a city. We know the grief and fear parents feel with a missing child today, but what of a time before Amber alerts and mass communication? Before even photographs to show and say, *"Have you seen this child?"*

Her husband, it seems, passed away, and she and her son must have worked together to make ends meet in their household. But in the wake of the religious fervor John the Baptist inspired, her son began to preach a message of religious conversion. For a short while he stayed close to home, but his mother did not want him to hold back on her account. At a wedding celebration, when he was about thirty, she quietly pushed him into full-time ministry work. In the months and years that followed, his opinions and deeds caused family controversies, and then larger controversies than that. He was often away. But she was near him, in Jerusalem, one spring when he was arrested on trumped-up charges. The presiding judge seemed reluctant to find him guilty, but bowed to political pressure. This woman watched her son undergo an excruciating death, unable to hold him as she once did, all those years before.

Mary received no adverse prenatal diagnosis for her child, as we did for Elizabeth, yet she received an adverse prognosis, a warning during her pregnancy that her child would be contradicted, and a sword would pierce her heart. (Luke 2:34-35). Mary's child was not born with a hole in his brain, like my daughter Elizabeth, but Mary saw his head wounded with the crown of thorns. (E.g. Matt. 27:29). The Blessed Mother did not live with a child bound to a wheelchair, but she lived with a child who would be bound to a cross.

God gave himself to the world through Mary. Of all the options he had, he gave himself to the world through the love of a parent. He knew how she would suffer. Her *Yes* to God was as much a *Yes* to the sufferings that were to come as it was to the joy. The two were inseparable. God chose this route—becoming a child, part of a family, with a human mother—knowing the hardship it would cause the one he loved. He needed Mary to be more than a mother. He needed Mary to be a model of love through suffering, so that we may turn our eyes to her in our need, meditating on her experience, and asking her to be with us as we walk with her son.

Walking with those who walk with Christ gives me hope, inspiration, and comfort. I can turn to St. Elizabeth and St. Thérèse, or Mother Teresa and the Mother of God, and know that I am not alone, that others have walked this path before me, and they are ready to help. But these saints and heroes are only aids, pointing always back to our mutual love—the Lord, Jesus Christ.

I would not withstand the challenges of raising Elizabeth if I were not able to walk with Christ, and with those who walk with him. I need something beyond myself and my family, to give context to the tough times within the family. I need these challenges to be just a tiny part of a much larger story, so this challenge matters both immensely for us, with everlasting implications, and very little, because other things matter far more, things I don't have to worry about, things someone far greater than me has handled already. I need to live in the absurd state of mind where I care deeply and passionately, without clinging to a desired outcome. I don't know how to maintain this perspective without believing in God, and a particular God at that.

I need God to be not simply a distant, fatherly figure, looking over us. I need him to be the ground of every atom of my being, every synapse of mind, and those of my wife and family, and those of the doctors and nurses and teachers and caregivers for Elizabeth. I am not God, and I don't need others to be God, but I need God to be the very foundation of being, as a playwright is the foundation of a performance on the stage. I need a God who is not simply an abstraction, a spiritual being, but one who allows me to say that he has shown us the way, through a flesh and blood example. I need to know that even in my worst times, he has been there before. He knows from experience what it is like.

I need a God who is not simply convenient, but a God of high standards, calling us to perfection, because otherwise I will make excuses about why I do not need to be the best version of myself. But I need a God of infinite mercy, because far too often I know I am not the best version of myself.

This is the God I find in Christianity: A God whose name is *I AM*, for he is the source and foundation of all that is. A God who entered history as man, and lived, and ate, and drank, and taught, and healed, and forgave, and suffered, and died, and rose again.

We pray with and for Elizabeth tonight. These are not perfect prayers. We are too often distracted by the children or proceed thoughtlessly through a routine. For some moments, though, I can steal away from the diversions of the world and peer into the significance of what I say. I can hold before my mind's eye each of my family members as we ask for God's blessings on them. I can invite my wife and children to ponder what we need, and what we have received, embracing the gifts with gratitude, and placing our petitions in faith before our God. I can stare at the heroes we have selected as our patrons and ask them to solicit God for aid on our behalf. By these prayers with my family, we move together day by day on this road of redemption, walking with those who walk with God.

Become the Ones Who Made It Through
Managing Medical Crises

Tonight, I lie again on a makeshift bed in the Charlottesville hospital, three feet from Elizabeth. A device, screwed to the front of her skull, reports her intracranial pressure in real time. With a bandage wrapped like a cone around the device, she seems to have a unicorn horn.

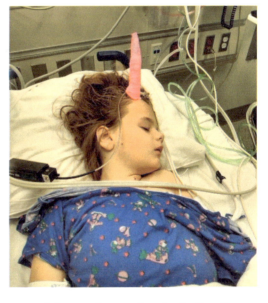

It has been a hell of a month. Elizabeth has depended on antinausea medication to keep down any food and drink. Multiple hospital visits ruled out the obvious causes for her vomiting, without providing answers. Often, at home, I woke before 5 a.m. to deliver a new dose of her medicine, while delaying as long as I could. If the morning dose wore off too soon, she would vomit in the evening. But when I delayed too long, she might not keep down the pill.

Meanwhile my wife proceeded through the thirty-ninth week of pregnancy with Philip, and then the fortieth. Every day was the day for delivery, until it wasn't. We had to balance Elizabeth's illness against my need to be available whenever Philip came. Yet every time I called the doctors about Elizabeth, they wanted her to return to the hospital, to rule out again what they ruled out before.

The call from Joyce finally came at forty-one weeks. Our nanny watched the girls while we were in the hospital. Philip's delivery went well, but Elizabeth lost ground over the weekend. I was back on the phone, trying to hold the pieces together, until the hospital discharged Joyce and Philip. Forty-five hours after my son's birth, six hours after we arrived home, I left my wife with our newborn and two daughters to take Elizabeth back to the emergency room.

The hospital had no bed for Elizabeth beyond the emergency department. Instead, after eighteen hours and a sleepless night, Elizabeth went to the operating room to receive this device on her skull. Yet even after the surgery, the hospital still had no room for her, until twenty-eight hours after we arrived. And so ended day two.

Day three I spent advocating for my daughter. Neurosurgery took the lead on the case, but I could not allow other medical teams simply to hope this pet theory from neurosurgery was correct. Nor could I let the neurosurgery team freely do as it thought best. After ten hours with the device, Elizabeth knocked it loose, and the team decided to remove it. They had enough data, they assured me, to see the pressure was in the low acceptable range. I argued they had nearly ten hours of Elizabeth lying down, where the pressure would be at its peak, and about five minutes of her upright, where it would be at its lowest. We needed to know more. Eventually, the doctors agreed, and reluctantly secured the device instead of removing it. By the end of the day, they decided the shunt was probably broken, and the pressures were too low, but they wanted to change the shunt setting again and continue the monitoring for another day. And so tonight, at the end of day four, they scheduled a shunt replacement surgery for tomorrow.

Meanwhile, after managing the kids each day, Joyce still must wrestle two girls into bed, and then wake up hourly to feed Philip.

Elizabeth was feeling ill again this afternoon and refused dinner. She ate a little at bedtime, after her antinausea pill. She was not restful, and started to vocalize. I could hear the exhausted parents of a two-week old child sharing the hospital room settling in to sleep between nighttime feedings, and I didn't want Elizabeth to keep them up. I gave my daughter melatonin. As sleep came to claim her, I went for a walk.

It was Thursday night in a college town, the week before classes, and my first time outside since Monday. The deliberate frivolity of college kids seeking an evening thrill brought me back to my own college days. I felt envy and emptiness. How I would love to lay aside the burden of caring for Elizabeth, and spend a night with good friends and no real concerns, believing that life lay at our feet for the taking. But did I really want that? Would I really want to give up all that life, and love, and suffering has taught me over the last fifteen years? My cup of life was so small in college it was easy to fill. If I felt emptiness in this month of tribulation, it is not because I have less in my life. I have a greater capacity. Still, I did feel empty, and my joyful college days seemed a lifetime ago.

I called Joyce, but she was exhausted and stressed and needed sleep. We said a quick good night. I was tired too, but sleep would not help. I tapped a long text to my sister, who knows how to hear without fixing things. I told her I wasn't worried about the surgery tomorrow, but the decision felt like a guess. The doctors were fixing something they could see that might be a problem, because they had nothing else to fix.

It took me time to find the words I wanted. I didn't need life to be easy, I wrote. Easy is not good for me. But I wanted now to be the person who made it through this.

Being is easy. *Becoming* is difficult. Yet as parents of special needs children, we are so often becoming. Maybe we are always becoming, but in times like this, the hill is steeper and our burden weighs heavier. Yet because we have walked this steep path so often, we can look back, and our progress is more apparent. When I was a college kid, enjoying my friends and wondering what life had in store, I was not the man who could do this. But I accepted the preparation, and here I am. That is some comfort, as the hill climbs in front of me.

Yet a few weeks ago, a doctor asked if Elizabeth was showing any signs of puberty. I told my wife I resign. I am not ready for that. That should be far away. *Far*, far away. *Unimaginably* far away. *Never-going-to-happen* far away. But it isn't. It lies just up the hill. I must become the man that is ready for it.

In times like this, we parents of special needs children either become the ones that made it through, or we shirk our duty, or we break. We will not shirk our duty. We may break someday, but we will not choose to break. The only path forward is becoming one that made it through.

Becoming that person doesn't mean we will do things perfectly. But G.K. Chesterton tells us if a thing is worth doing, it's worth doing badly. A man in love may write poor love letters, but doing it badly is better than not doing it, or getting another to do it for him. Children follow this lesson well. They sing badly, but they sing, even in public. They paint badly, but they paint. If it's worth doing, it's worth doing badly. This doesn't excuse poor efforts, but measures what's really important. And raising our child despite the difficulties is worth doing, even when we do it badly.

We parents of special needs children can inventory what we often do badly. My family does church badly. Elizabeth grows bored and rakes her ankle braces against her wheelchair, clicks her heals together, and pounds them back into her chair, to start again. The music of *rake, clip, thump, rake, click, thump* interrupts the priest's homily. Meanwhile, my two-year-old rediscovers the passageway beneath the pew to the freedom that lies beyond. We pull her back by the ankle or grab her as she escapes. Our five-year-old asks us about the great mystery she associates with the mass: *"Daddy, can we get donuts?"* Sitting in the wheelchair-accessible pew near the front, we distract everyone. And now we will have a newborn. Still, we worship God and teach our children to worship God, as we can. We do church badly, but we do church.

We parent badly sometimes. Elizabeth's needs make it difficult to teach my middle daughter to ride a bike or to fit in that eye appointment for my youngest daughter. The television is on too much, and we don't have the one-on-one time we would like with each child. But our children have three siblings. We parent badly, but we parent.

And we manage Elizabeth's condition badly. Today, our insurance company called to offer us a nurse care coordinator. In other words, we are costing them so much money, paying a nurse to bug us may be cheaper. I declined. We can't seem to manage all our care coordinators. Most of the mail we receive for Elizabeth we leave unopened, knowing it is probably just paperwork. Joyce can't remember Elizabeth's medication dosing, and I don't know how to contact her bus driver. But we have given her seven years of life. We manage Elizabeth's condition badly, but together we do it.

We special parents do things badly, but eventually we become the ones who made it through. Our burden seems absurd to those who stand outside. I am often astounded by what other special needs parents endure, just as they are astounded by our story. Our mutual admiration shows how far we have already come.

To make it through, though, we must grow our coping skills. Connecting with others helps in these emergencies. Generous friends have blessed Joyce with assistance this week, while Elizabeth and I are away. Meanwhile, I find support from other parents of special needs children. They can reach past the clichés, to offer true emotional support. I exchanged messages with a classmate caring for her special needs daughter at a hospital in Cincinnati. Another friend, whose son has a genetic anomaly, shared a video of a father mimicking the different characters you meet in the NICU: the rule-abiding travel nurse, the resident who doesn't know the answer, the carefree surgeon. All week, now, I have been silently labeling my providers. These small acts have meant so much to me.

Be attentive to your emotional energy. This week I am anchored to a room, low on sleep, far from my family, missing the first week of my son's life, acting as caregiver, advocate, and decision-maker for my daughter. I need to eliminate, for a time, things that deplete energy from my reserves. As an introvert, constant updates to well-meaning family and friends exhaust me. And so I limit my communications, so I can be what I need to be for my daughter and my family. I find things that will engage me, but not require deliberation or substantial concentration, so that I can save my energy for Elizabeth. It works for me, and in moments like this, what works matters.

Be merciful to yourself. During a prolonged crisis, it's easy to slip into imperfect behaviors. But some are innocent indulgences we should tolerate for a time. The self-discipline we ordinarily exert may require more emotional energy than we can afford. And if we make a mistake, we own it, but don't disregard the extraordinary context of the mistake in the self-critique.

Some of my conservative friends resist enrolling their special needs children in Medicaid, but I encourage them to do so, if the children qualify. Medicaid allows me to care for my daughter in moments of crisis without being concerned about the financial detriment to my family. Medicaid is far, far, far from a perfect system. But when a single MRI may cost thousands, and the doctors rely on MRIs, and X-rays, and CAT scans, and emergency departments, and surgeries, and multiple daily medications to keep my daughter alive, I bless God that I don't have to factor costs into my analysis of what care to pursue for my daughter. All the extra items I need for Elizabeth—from a wheelchair accessible van, to home modifications, to an in-home nanny, to time off of work—already factor heavily into the budget, even after Medicaid coverage.

We must also learn how to work with doctors. Modern medicine upholds the ideal of patient autonomy, including the right to accept or refuse care. But the decision maker must often rely on the wisdom of the doctor. Trusting doctors makes their job easier, and so they encourage it, even acting as though their recommendations are the decision. If the patient seeks explanations or raises objections, the doctors may proffer only the information that supports the doctor's plan and perspective. Young residents seem particularly prone to selling their ideas, likely because they do not have adequate experience to explain the reasons and alternatives, but they want to appear confident and competent.

We must be ready to insist on our right to be the decision maker, and we must be confident we know more about the particulars of our child than the doctors. They are the experts as to the condition and the body. You are the expert as to your child. You know better the routine that keeps your child's health and wellbeing in balance. You know her moods and what soothes her. You know how she reacts to medication and treatment. They may deal with a thousand similar cases, but you deal with this case. They will tend to treat your child as an ordinary case. You know how your child is unique. They review charts and records. You have lived experience.

Doctors approach diagnostics by asking *What is most probable?* This involves guesswork for unusual conditions or unusual patients. Yet collecting information takes time, and the symptoms may demand immediate action. And so, physicians generally prioritize treating any symptoms that pose imminent or serious risks, and then focus on causes that can be tested, treated, or which pose the gravest and most immediate threats. They may discount conditions that cannot be tested or treated, or which are unlikely, or which are not immediately threatening. But treating symptoms may impede a diagnosis, by suppressing information or creating false flags.

Press the doctors to articulate what they are seeing and the reasons for their recommendations. *What is the biggest risk right now? Why? How can it be treated? What are the pros, cons, probabilities, and alternatives? Have you considered the side effects of the treatment, or possible drug interactions? What can cause these symptoms? Which causes can be tested and treated? How? What are the pros, cons, and alternatives of each test or treatment? How long will the test take to generate information? What can we expect to see if your theory is correct? And if it is wrong? How will the treatment of the symptoms affect the test? What avenues can we pursue simultaneously? If we can't pursue them simultaneously, which do we prioritize, and why?* Through these questions and a hundred more, you can work with the doctors to build a plan of care. Typically, if the doctor sees in you a skilled and cooperative advocate and decision maker, he will more readily collaborate with you.

Be patient if the doctors do not have answers. Medicine is not magic. It is a science with more questions than answers, and children with special needs often stretch the science. The condition may pass before an answer comes. And sometimes, there is no answer. How many symptoms earn the label *idiopathic?* What other profession uses such a long word to say *"We don't know why"?*

Presume you are a critical hub for keeping different medical teams on the same page. One team's action may hurt the treatment plan as a whole. Since you are the decision maker—the last barrier before a team acts—you should know how the decision will affect the overall plan, and this requires you to know how each plan fits together.

Look for signs that a doctor is overconfident in his theory, or that he expects some other team will find a solution. Doctors sometime fall into the traps of *I see it, so it must be the cause*, or *My colleague is confident, so he must be right*. When a doctor finds a workable theory within his specialty, even if it is improbable, he may try to take over the case. Meanwhile, other teams may stand back, waiting in the wings instead of working simultaneously or collaboratively with the lead team. Ask early and often what other teams should be involved, and ask to see those teams.

When dealing with medical professionals, remember to love fiercely. The medical industry is bureaucratic. It relies on protocols. These protocols save lives. But there comes a time—quite often in fact—when bureaucracy and protocols obstruct care. Some righteous anger may be appropriate. But be cautious. A medical provider has great power to leave a permanent stain on your records if he feels slighted, and he will get away with it. Advocacy with a collaborative attitude usually works better than anger with doctors, and persistence usually works better than shouting with insurance companies. There are complaint processes available, but they usually take time, so don't allow them to distract you in the middle of caring for your child in a crisis. The greatest power you have in the medical context, though, is the power to say *No*. You can withdraw your consent if you need. If a technician seems to be doing more harm than good in getting a blood draw, tell him in clear terms that he is to stop right now. If a doctor orders a medication that you do not want administered, tell the nurse that you need to speak with him before she administers it, and tell him your concerns. You generally have the right to say no. Use it wisely.

Still, connect with the doctors, nurse practitioners, and the nurses. A human connection both eases the advocacy and enlightens the day. Invariably I ask if it has been a busy shift, as this gently turns attention away to their concerns. I try to find the point of connection, particularly with the nursing staff, as they know best the little ways to make a big impact on the care experience.

We must also prepare for the possibility that the crisis will continue for the long-term. *Who will be with the child? Who will be with the other children? How will we afford the bills?* We won't have answers to all these questions, but it's worthwhile to think about the questions.

Elizabeth's condition may have no short-term cure. I am not guaranteed to make it through this on my timetable. In fact, it may have no long-term cure. We may not return to her previous level of health. But I still must become the person who can rise to the needs of my family, come what may. I must find the coping skills, the resources, the connections, and the habits and patterns of life to deal, however imperfectly, with the crises.

I take comfort in the fact, though, that God gave me *this child* for his glory, and God gave *me* this child for his glory. When I am caring for Elizabeth in her time of need, I am where I am supposed to be. We don't always know what God is asking of us, but in times like this, I do. I am supposed to be *here*.

Think of the path *Abram* walked to become *Abraham*. Think of the path *Saul* walked to become *Paul*. We are meant in life to be transformed in faith, transformed in Christ. For many, they have no anchor for their transformation—no focal point given by God for that change. But caring for this child of God, this image of God's glory, is a key to your transformation in Christ. He will change you through your cooperation in this project of love.

This week, on Sunday afternoon, a Eucharistic minister from the local parish made his rounds in the hospital, offering communion to the Catholics. He asked to meet Elizabeth, and I told him a little of her story. He looked at me and told me compassionately of his special needs daughter, whom he and his wife raised for four and a half years. And like so many who have walked this path, he told me she was his greatest blessing. We prayed together, and he gave me the Body of Christ—Christ, who went all the way to the point of death to be with us in our brokenness, and who, by his Resurrection, became the one who made it through.

I write this while still sitting on the makeshift bed in the hospital, a week after we arrived in the emergency department. Elizabeth turned a corner this morning. She did not show us her signs of nausea, and she seemed eager to eat. For the first time in three weeks, she has gone six hours over the scheduled administration of her antinausea drug without becoming sick. It seems we are on the cusp of making it through. Tomorrow, I hope, we will go home, to be with my wife, my daughters, and my new son. But for today, Elizabeth and I are still becoming the ones who made it through.

Lesson Twelve

Be Grateful
Recognizing God's Gifts

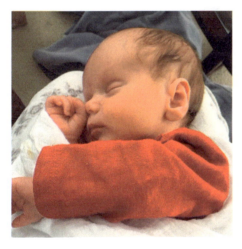

Seven and a half years ago, in the NICU, I stared with wonder at this beautiful child, marveling at the smallest of things, like the way she clutched tiny wires from the monitors between her toes. I sat there for hours, just to be with her.

I never changed a diaper before that day in the NICU. But here was a child I would raise. She was my responsibility. My wife and I would name her Elizabeth, and that name would be hers through all eternity.

My wife chose to love me, and I chose to love my wife. We each made that choice, because we found in the other the foundation for a life and a family. But this was different. I felt no sense of choice in my love of Elizabeth, and I desired no choice. I wanted nothing but to love this beautiful child.

We did not know, at that time, the functional limitations Elizabeth would face. We would learn within a week that the congenital brain malformation affected her speech cortex. We noticed the signs of excessive pressure on her brain within five weeks. A doctor disclosed her visual impairment within months. The developmental delay became obvious by six months. Epilepsy appeared near the end of her first year. A doctor diagnosed cerebral palsy after a year and a half.

But Elizabeth wove her way into our life, and into our hearts. We watched as she developed a personality: Introverted, but without fear of strangers. Cunning in her resistance of things she dislikes. Delighting in simple pleasures of cuddles, her angel doll, savory foods, and music. Incredibly tolerant of pain and discomfort, but feisty and strong when she felt we were not listening. We started to notice how she engaged the world differently. She would rarely look at us directly. She conveyed much through her subtle expressions, gestures, and vocalization. Everything would go to her mouth so she could explore it with her tongue. She liked to dance in her wheelchair and make noise with her hands and feet.

I love the little moments with my daughter, like the way she will press my hand to her cheek as she sucks her thumb, and will squeeze tight and hold me there if I give the slightest sign of pulling away. Like the way she lifts her eyebrows and her gaze, and then sits up straight, when she hears a song she enjoys. Or the way she senses in an instant whether the food I offer, or the medicine I have to administer, will be unacceptable, leading her to clench her lips and her cheeks unequivocally.

This is not the life I would have chosen for myself, if it was offered to me years ago. When I promised to have and to hold my wife for better or for worse, I thought we would have babies, and those babies would become adults, and the adults would eventually leave our home. I did not expect a child who would need my love and care as long as we both shall live.

This is not the life I would have chosen for myself. I grew up in a family that loved road trips and sightseeing. We enjoyed camping and spending Sundays swimming and mini-golfing at the park. We spent our weekends gardening. I sometimes dream of getting back to these things, but the practical challenges of Elizabeth's needs and conditions intrude. Every plan must be checked against the feasibility of a wheelchair, a safe bed, and diaper changes in public facilities.

This is not the life I would have chosen for myself. By every objective description, this life seems a drudgery for the uninitiated. Would you choose changing diapers for your girl all her life? Of lifting her daily from her bed to her wheelchair and back again? Of never hearing her speak your name, or say *"I love you"*?

But relationships are not what we plan them to be. They are not the activities we do. They are not captured by objective descriptions. Relationships must be experienced before they can be enjoyed. *Taste and see that the LORD is good.* (Ps. 34:8). Taste and see. This is not the life I would have chosen for myself, and I recognize that now with regret. I simply could not have imagined what a small man I was, compared to the man this relationship would lead me to be. I could not have imagined how a little girl, with so many limitations, would show me the boundless capacities of my love.

This is not the life I would have chosen, but in fact, I did choose the possibility of this life. I stood before God and my community and said, "For better, for worse, for richer, for poorer, in sickness and health." I made the commitment not only to my wife, but to the family we would raise. In the Small Room, in a distant hospital, I felt that commitment challenged, but my wife and I again chose to accept the unknown. *For better, for worse, for richer, for poorer, in sickness and health.*

I am incredibly, deeply, richly grateful to God for giving me Elizabeth. Grateful beyond imagination. Grateful beyond words. I cannot imagine how life could be better without her. I cannot imagine how *I* could be better without her. God has given me the gift of a special needs child in my life.

The world might call her condition a tragedy. The world might measure her against the norm of a healthy child. And yet I cannot help but wish the world might taste the joy I have in loving this child. It seems, in making that wish, I would want more children to suffer such conditions. All I can say is *God's will be done.* I do not think such love is possible apart from this intimate encounter with special needs. I know I would not have understood without this being my daughter. We need to embrace these children, every one of them, recognizing in these children the invitation to a relationship of inestimable worth.

For many families, the challenge of raising a child with severe special needs would be overwhelming. Financially and emotionally, caring for someone with special needs comes with a heavy cost. We need to support these families. Our human condition carries the certainty that without eugenic programs, some of us will have special needs, even severe special needs. The greater the burden on the special needs family, the less the family will contribute its other special gifts to society. No social welfare or community aid program will eliminate the burden of doctors' visits and therapies and medication regimens and managing caregivers. And they don't have to. But no Christian principle justifies placing this burden on the family alone, just because the child happens to belong to the family.

I am grateful that God has not asked me, so far, to accept a challenge beyond my strength. Or rather, I thank God that he has given me abundance to meet our needs. He has blessed my wife and me each with a good job, flexibility, and support. I must not take this for granted, for God may call me at any time to a greater level of sacrifice. I must accept these comforts, this present margin of safety, as a gift, without becoming dependent on it or clinging to it.

We cannot be grateful without recognizing the good things in our lives *didn't have to be*. We must see the good *as good*, and see the good *as contingent*. Gratitude presumes things are good, and things could be different. But often we struggle to see the good through the distractions and the suffering, and we forget that what has happened didn't have to happen, and what is commonplace may still be extraordinary.

I am grateful for Elizabeth's facial expressions, her vocalizations, her gestures, and her signs, because each of these helps me to connect with her world. Despite our thousand ways to communicate with one another, communication itself—the ability to encounter the mind of another—is a remarkable gift.

I am grateful for Elizabeth's love of music. This path would be so much harder without this passion. I can offer her music when I cannot be available, physically or emotionally, to entertain her. I can raise my voice in song to let her know when I am near, and to calm her in times of distress. I can leave the radio playing through the night, as a nightlight for my blind child, until we can be with her in the morning.

I am grateful for the balance we call Elizabeth's health, because I have experienced so many days where I thought the best we could do was not this good. I have also experienced so many days when good things changed for the worse, and I would be bound for an indefinite stay with her at the hospital. I am grateful for the doctors and the nurses who have cared for her, and who have guided me in parenting this child.

I am grateful for all those who have helped Elizabeth, and who have helped Joyce and me—family, friends, teachers, and strangers. Our nanny, in particular, has been a second mother to these children, giving the best part of her energy to raising them. She has endured the injuries Elizabeth sometimes inflicts, and she has strained to lift, and carry, and cuddle with Elizabeth. And she has earned Elizabeth's love, and Joyce's and my eternal appreciation.

I am grateful Elizabeth has siblings. Seeing my five-year-old and two-year-old take care of Elizabeth—pushing her chair, feeding her, holding her hand and showing her affection—gives me hope they will encounter others, *all others*, in love. I look forward to my son's encounter with his biggest sister.

I am grateful for my wife—my companion on this journey. We have been tested together, and our marriage is stronger. This is the place I am meant to be in life, and I am meant to share it with her.

This list may seem almost cliché. But I am surprised I feel genuine gratitude simply for the emotional vulnerability Elizabeth has brought into my life. The right word, the right thought, or an image of sacrificial suffering can rekindle instantly the sense of the Small Room, or walking the hospital ward all night before the first surgery, or seeing the angel doll in the midnight reflection, or watching Elizabeth seize in the emergency room. I do not regret the experiences, for they help me to encounter others in their struggles and fears, to meet them in their moments of need. Through these memories, I am more alive to the world, and to the suffering of others. And in this suffering, I see saints in the making.

We men so often suppress our feelings, usually as part of being in control. We strive for emotional invulnerability. There is a time and place to suppress emotions. In an emergency, our vocation, especially we men, is to act deliberately and prudently, even at the cost of our wellbeing. Sometimes that means suppressing our emotional vulnerability. But our emotions empower us to quickly prioritize our values, and so our emotional wellbeing is central to our moral wellbeing. I am not ashamed of strong emotions. I am not ashamed of tears. The urge to cry is our mind adjusting to a new reality, and that is okay. Harness the emotions as a partner and guide for the intuition.

Christ shows us the priority of gratitude time and time again. In the multiplication of loaves and fishes, in the institution of the Eucharist at the Last Supper, and in the breaking of bread with the disciples on the road to Emmaus, he takes the bread and gives thanks, before distribution. (Matt. 14:19, 15:36, 26:26-27; Mark 6:41, 8:6, 14:22-23; Luke 9:16, 22:19, 24:30; John 6:11; 1 Cor. 11:24). John recognizes the central role of this gratitude, describing the location for the multiplication of the loaves as *"the place where they had eaten the bread when the Lord gave thanks."* (John 6:23).

Similarly, in raising Lazarus, Christ speaks a prayer of gratitude. *"Father, I thank you for hearing me. I know that you always hear me; but because of the crowd here I have said this, that they may believe that you sent me."* And then he commands, *"Lazarus, come out!"* (John 11:41-43). These are mysterious words. The prayer preempts the accusation that Christ raises Lazarus by evil powers. He's been accused of such things before. (Mark 3:22). But the open appeal to God before the miracle makes God a witness to the display of power, and the crowd knows God would not allow this man to then perform a life-restoring act by the power of Satan. Still, this does not explain why Christ chose *to give thanks.* Any prayer to the Father would do.

But Christ is showing us that a prayer of gratitude has particular power, because it credits God, and not our action. Christ is showing that gratitude should fundamentally shape our outlook on the created world. It should be the context of all our petitions.

St. Paul writes, *"Rejoice always. Pray without ceasing. In all circumstances give thanks, for this is the will of God for you in Christ Jesus."* (1 Thes. 5:16-18). In all circumstances, give thanks. Every circumstance presents good that didn't have to be. Life itself is always an unnecessary good. Relationships with others are always an unnecessary good.

If we want gratitude to shape our outlook, if we want to give thanks in all circumstances, if we want gratitude to be the context of our prayers of petition, gratitude must become more than just an emotion. We must habitually notice the unnecessary goodness in the created order. This lifts our spirits and readies us to receive God's gifts. It moves us from *fear and anxiety* to *possibility and abundance*. Fear shuts down our creative thinking, obscuring the path God laid before us. Responding with gratitude drives away fear, and opens the imagination to our full potential, and more importantly, to God's full potential in the moment.

We can develop the habit of gratitude by seeing suffering as ordinary, and comfort and solace as extraordinary. We don't deserve a pain-free existence. We don't deserve a stress-free existence. Our comforts are gifts to be celebrated. Our knowledge is a gift to be celebrated. Our relationships are gifts from God to be celebrated.

This habit of gratitude requires us to relinquish control. We must embrace our true vulnerability, for in recognizing without fear our vulnerability, we prepare ourselves to accept the unnecessary good with a grateful heart. It bears repeating: *Vulnerability, not control, teaches us gratitude*—the ability to delight in what we have, and in the relationships those things represent, because we know they did not have to be part of our life.

Elizabeth's vulnerability, and the vulnerability of our family, constantly remind me to be grateful. Elizabeth should have died years ago, with a brain crushed by the cerebrospinal fluid accumulating within her skull. But God gave mankind a way to manage that pressure. The prolonged seizure I saw in the emergency department should be Elizabeth's daily struggle, but God inspired a team to develop a drug to keep those seizures at bay. Even the pain of transitions, and the limitations of her mobility, would be so much greater without the wheelchair and other equipment God gave man the power to create. And so I give thanks to God, and I give thanks for the men and women whose names I will never know, who cooperated with God's grace to make this life with Elizabeth possible. And I thank God for giving me Elizabeth to teach me vulnerability and gratitude.

Gratitude should not become generic. It should be focused, as much as possible, on the particulars. It should not be simply, *"Lord, I thank you for a good time with my daughter,"* but rather, *"Lord, I thank you for the opportunity to hold my child today. I thank you for her excitement when I sang her favorite song. I thank you for the joy I felt in seeing her smile and dance."* The more particular we are, the more we can reap the benefits of gratitude. This is so because God works through particulars. He works through *specific moments*, and *particular items*, and *distinct actions*, and *individual relationships*. This is sometimes called the scandal of particularity. Why was Mary selected to give birth to Jesus? Well, God gets to choose the particular, and often it is not the particular moment, or item, or action, or relationship we would have chosen. For we think as man thinks, and not as God thinks. (Cf. Matt. 16:23).

In our human frailty, some of us will have special needs. And some of us will be the caregivers of those with special needs. For all the joy and suffering involved, we who have been chosen for this lot in life experience the scandal of particularity. We did *nothing* to deserve this. And we did nothing *to deserve this*. God selected us, and that is his prerogative. I, for my part, am grateful.

Last weekend, our parish celebrated a mass for our Special Blessings ministry, our support group for parents of special needs children. The coordinator asked me to lector. We used the reading for the day, but through God's blessing, the reading came from the first chapter of St. Paul's first letter to the Corinthians.

> *Consider your own calling, brothers and sisters.*
> *Not many of you were wise by human standards,*
> *not many were powerful,*
> *not many were of noble birth.*
> *Rather, God chose the foolish of the world to shame the wise,*
> *and God chose the weak of the world to shame the strong,*
> *and God chose the lowly and despised of the world,*
> *those who count for nothing,*
> *to reduce to nothing those who are something,*
> *so that no human being might boast before God.*
> *It is due to him that you are in Christ Jesus,*
> *who became for us wisdom from God,*
> *as well as righteousness, sanctification, and redemption,*
> *so that, as it is written,*
> *"Whoever boasts, should boast in the Lord."* (1 Cor. 1:26-31).

Reading this passage through my own experience, I stand accused. In humility, I must say I was wise by human standards. I pursued training in the law, graduating near the top of my class, with honors and accolades. I have built a worldly reputation as a stalwart litigator of civil rights and constitutional law. But the greatest lessons I learned in this life have come through a little girl who cannot speak, who can hardly see, who cannot walk. She is the foolish of the world, by any objective standard. She is the weak of the world by any true measure. She is the lowly and despised, and she reduces me to nothing. I did not deserve to father Elizabeth. I deserved nothing so grand. That was entirely the gracious work of our Lord. I am convinced she will be given a higher place in heaven through her union with Christ than I will ever see. When I stand at the final judgment, I could say, *"But look at the cases I won. Look at the good I have done with the law."* Or I can say, *"Dear Lord, by your grace, I was the father of Elizabeth."* I know which case I would prefer to plead.

Some will look at my child and wonder, *"Why would a loving God do this?"* I look at my child and say, *"What a loving God to give me her!"*

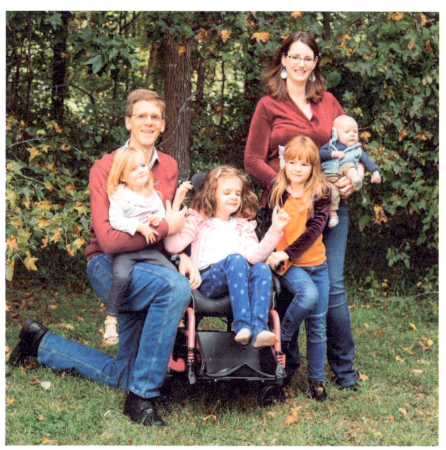

ABOUT THE AUTHOR

Andrew T. Bodoh is the father of four beautiful children, and the undeserving husband of his wonderful wife Joyce. Together, they live in Fredericksburg, Virginia, worshiping at St. Mary of the Immaculate Conceptions Catholic Church.

Andrew is a litigation attorney, serving as the senior associate for the firm of Thomas H. Roberts and Associates, P.C., in Richmond, Virginia. He specializes in civil rights and Constitutional law.

Made in United States
Cleveland, OH
21 April 2025

16283756R00070